COMBAT
Foot Pain

BY KARIN V. DRUMMOND, DC

COMBAT
FOOT PAIN

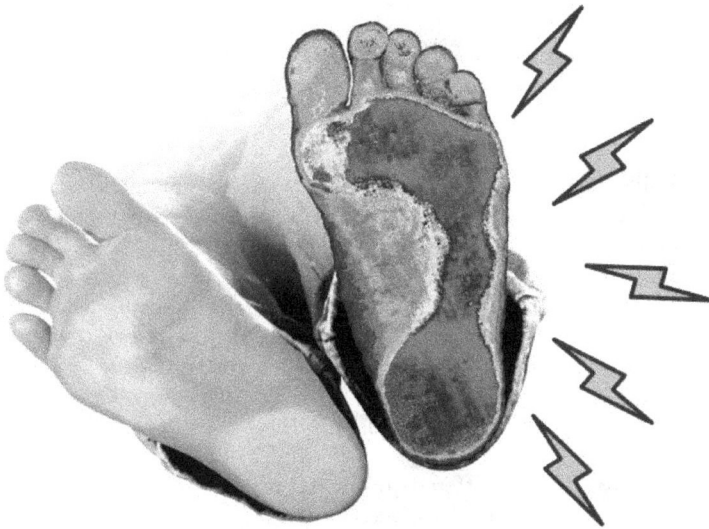

COMBAT DIS-EASE SERIES

BOOK 10

A chiropractor's advice
for those who suffer from
plantar fasciitis, bunions, heel pain,
Morton's Neuroma, cramps, and more

BY KARIN V. DRUMMOND, DC

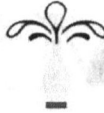

Published by Blooming Ink Publishing, LLC
4712 East State Road 46
Bloomington, IN 47401

Copyright ©2017 by Karin Drummond, DC
Cover art Copyright © 2018 by Drummond Chiropractic, LLC
Published in 2018

FIRST EDITION

ISBN: 978-1-943753-21-5

Library of Congress Number: 2016921488

Combat Dis-Ease Series 10

This book is dedicated to my patients and anyone who can benefit from reading my books.

Acknowledgments

Stephanie Smith, MT, for her input on cupping and Gua Sha
Jennifer Stone, BS, LAc, for her input on acupuncture and Gua Sha
Dr. Stanley Stanbridge, Chiropractic Physician and inventor of the
    Rapid Release Technology
Kip May Photography for my image on my book covers.
PenciLDesigns for designing my book covers.
Vicki Adang for her editing skills.
Dawn Galbraith, Senior Vic President of Foot Levelers for the permission to use Foot Leveler images
Dan Sweeney for supplying the images needed from Foot Levelers.

A Special Thank You To

Dr. Tim Maggs, Chiropractic Physician and founder of CPOYA™ (Concerned Parents of Young Athletes™).
    To learn more about how CPOYA practitioners examine young athletes and educate them on how to perform better and prevent injury, visit cpoya.com.

And thank you to countless others…

**This book is
my message in a bottle
in the sea of misinformation.**

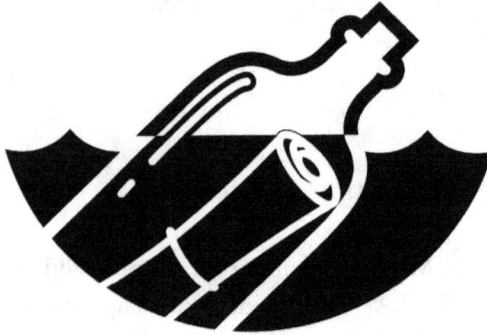

Other books by Dr. Karin Drummond:
- **Top Seven Ways to Combat the Effects of Sitting**
- **Combat Slouching**
- **Combat Headaches**
- **Combat Irritable Bowels**
- **Whiplash: More Than Just Neck Pain**
- **Whiplash to Wellness: A Chiropractor's Journey**
- **Combat Jaw Pain**
- **Combat Neck Pain**
- **Combat Low Back Pain**

Upcoming books
- **Combat Insomnia**
- **Release Your Weight**
- and more…

Preface

Dear reader,

I assume that because you bought this book, you or a loved one is suffering from some form of foot pain. Rest assured, I am writing this book for you.

Because I love to run, I have suffered episodic foot pain and leg cramps. Before enrolling in chiropractic college, I tried many treatments that failed. During chiropractic college, I finally found what worked for me. In the eighteen years since graduation, I have treated my patients' foot pain and have further differentiated which treatments work for certain ailments, those that don't work, and those that do more harm than good—all of which I disclose in this book.

Now it is not just my patients who will benefit from my knowledge. Reading this book will help those who suffer from foot pain so they can become more collaborative with their healthcare providers to determine possible causes, treatments to consider, and advice on how to get better.

We are all individuals with unique conditions and needs, so I advise that you seek the help of a professional for guidance before following the advice in this book.

I sincerely wish you and/or your loved one wellness and a speedy recovery.

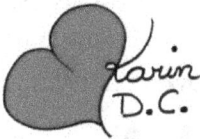

Karin
D.C.

Karin Drummond, D.C.

Dr. Karin's Definition of Dis-ease

Dis-ease results when a person is under prolonged stress, independent of whether the stressor is physical or mental. Simply, it is a state of agitation and non-relaxation.

The human body evolved to handle physical stress: You either survive or you die. For example, if you get attacked by a tiger, your body automatically goes through steps to decide whether to fight or flee. Your adrenaline kicks in, activated by your fight-or-flight sympathetic nervous system.

Blood flows out of your internal organs and into your arms and legs. This rerouting of energy and blood gives you extra strength and endurance, and decreases the amount of blood loss you would experience from your organs if you were to be wounded. Your primitive brain controls all of this automatically; you don't even think about it. Your only job is to act and survive.

The primitive brain cannot tell the difference between a mental and a physical stressor. Its reaction is the same: to prepare your body for fight or flight. But if your stressor is the result of your job or an argument with a loved one, the primitive brain's fight-or-flight response is disproportional to the threat of the stressor. Your body is prepared to move, but instead you sit, tense. This is unhealthy over time because the lymphatic system (the body's sewage system) requires movement to drain the metabolic waste out of your tissues.

The most-distant parts of our body that need to be drained are the feet. To make matters worse, the drainage in the feet

This can lead to foot pain!

typically has to work against gravity. Impairment of this drainage can lead to swelling of the lower extremities.

If the muscles stay tense, they not only prevent lymphatic drainage, but also impair the blood flow to the very muscles being contracted. These constantly contracting muscles produce metabolic waste (lactic acid) and need the oxygen-filled blood to be able to contract; yet they are blocking the very flow of fluids that brings in their nutrients and drains their waste. Sitting while you are tense and stressed out is unhealthy over time because it leads to the buildup of toxins in the body. This is one reason why stressed people tend to be tender to touch, especially in the feet.

Prolonged stress leads to adrenal fatigue; if you need a boost of energy, your body just doesn't have it to give to you. Your digestive system suffers from the diminished blood supply

This can lead to muscle cramps in the lower extremities!

(because the fight-or-flight response has diverted blood away from internal organs). Then your appetite changes as you become deficient in nutrients within the intestines, leading to either weight gain or excessive weight loss, neither of which are healthy.

Your blood pressure also goes up as a result of oversupplying blood to your extremities for the anticipated fight or flight. Over time, your arteries harden from being under such high pressure in a low-nutrient environment.

Eventually, your body starts deteriorating, becoming more susceptible to sickness. Every day your body fights viruses, bacteria, and fungi as well as mutations in a few of your one hundred trillion cells. It starts to lose these battles when weakened by stress, thus becoming more susceptible to colds, allergies, flu viruses, infections, cancer, and other grave diseases.

This can make you vulnerable to fungal infections and warts!

Stress is the number-one cause of death; it's just given names like heart attack, cancer, stroke, suicide, etc.

This book addresses the symptoms specifically of the foot, which is a sign of being in a dis-eased state. This book offers advice on how to break this vicious cycle of foot pain. The stress of pain leads to a state of "dis-ease," which in turn leads to physical disease and, potentially, an early death.

BE AT EASE, AVOID DIS-EASE!

Table of Contents

Contents

Chapter 1: WARNING SIGNS THAT YOUR FOOT PAIN MAY BE A SIGN OF A MORE SERIOUS CONDITION

BEFORE I REVEAL how to cure your foot pain, first I must inform you when it is imperative to seek medical attention. It would be irresponsible of me to say you could self-treat when, in fact, your foot pain is a symptom of an underlying disease that needs medical treatment, if not immediate care.

Our feet are the parts of our body that are the most distant from the major organs in our torso, so if we are in a dis-eased state or have a disease that is taxing our health, the problem is often expressed in some way in the feet. At times, I have detected a patient is unwell just by inspecting their hands and feet.

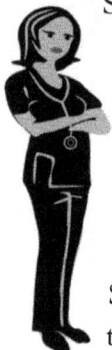

So, look out for any new foot symptoms. If the frequency of the symptom increases or if it is more intense than usual and is accompanied by numbness, tingling, weakness, or visible changes to the foot, seek immediate medical attention! It could be a sign of a more serious condition.

Seek immediate medical attention if you have any of these symptoms:

- Tingling, numbness, and susceptibility to foot infections; could be a sign of uncontrolled diabetes, which can cause nerve and tissue damage.
- Strange sensations in the feet, with weakness and fatigue; could be a sign of a vitamin deficiency.
    - Vitamin B deficiency causes anemia, in which the blood has a reduced ability to deliver oxygen to the tissues. This typically affects the most distal extremities first, like the feet. It can affect gait because the nerves aren't getting enough oxygen, making it difficult to walk (causing you to stagger). Extreme cases affect the liver, causing yellowing of the skin (jaundice).
    - Iron deficiency causes another form of anemia, which can lead to cold feet, brittle nails, and other symptoms (fatigue, headaches, chest pain, etc.).
- Swelling with pitting edema and waxy-looking skin. Pitting edema is a condition in which when you press on the skin, it leaves an indentation that is slow to fill back in. This can be a sign of deep vein thrombosis

14

(DVT), where a clot limits the venous drainage of the lower leg. The clot can break off and travel through the bloodstream until it gets trapped in the smaller vessels of the lungs, blocking blood flow, which is life threatening. DVT is diagnosed by ultrasound and needs medical treatment.

- Foot pain with numbness or tingling; could be a sign of neurotoxemia (poisoning of the nerves by medications).
- Swelling; could be a sign of a heart condition (cardiovascular disease).
- Cramping and impaired healing (wounds heal slowly), could be a sign of peripheral artery disease (PAD), which is can be a symptom of diabetes.
- Painfully cold feet; could be a sign of Raynaud's disease (risk of frostbite because it affects the blood supply to the hands and feet).
- Sharp, burning pain in the joints; could be a sign of rheumatoid arthritis or other autoimmune diseases, like psoriasis, which can cause holes, grooves or ridges in toe nails. Such autoimmune diseases attack tissues like skin, nails, joints, including those found in the feet.
- Extreme sharp pain; may be a sign of gout (uric acid deposits feel like shards of glass in the joint). If you have gout, you have a higher risk of kidney stones.
- Severe skin dryness; could indicate thyroid problems.
- Foot drop; can be a sign of a neurologic, back, or leg condition and needs to be examined immediately before permanent nerve damage can occur.
- Tiny red lines under the toenail, which are actually broken blood vessels; could be a sign of endocarditis

(an infection of the heart that can be fatal).

- Severe swelling where the foot looks like a club; can be caused by decreased vascular resistance as more blood flow to the fingertips and toes, causing them to swell. This is a sign of lung, heart, or intestinal disease or cancer.
- Nails that are spoon shaped (can hold a drop of water on them); can be a sign of iron deficiency or hemochromatosis (too much iron), Raynaud's disease (mentioned earlier), or lupus (another autoimmune disease).
- A straight dark line from your cuticle to the edge of your nail; could be caused by a mole, fungus, melanoma (skin cancer), or a side effect of a medication.
- A sudden high arch; could be nerve damage or a neuromuscular condition (i.e. Charcot-Marie-Tooth, which is an inherited disorder that damages peripheral nerves).
- Clawing of the toes; may be a sign of a neurologic condition.

Healthy feet are a sign of good overall health; painful feet can be a sign of other conditions.

Now that we have discussed symptoms of the feet that should be checked out immediately, let's look at the biomechanical causes of foot pain. Future chapters discuss treatment options for such conditions.

Chapter 2: ANATOMY OF THE FOOT

TO UNDERSTAND YOUR FOOT PAIN, you need to understand the foot. The structure of the foot is an engineering marvel. The foot has to be strong enough to withstand your weight, yet flexible enough to absorb the shock of high-impact activities.

The foot's arches hold weight, similar to how an arch supports the weight of a bridge over a span of space, as shown in Figure 2-1.

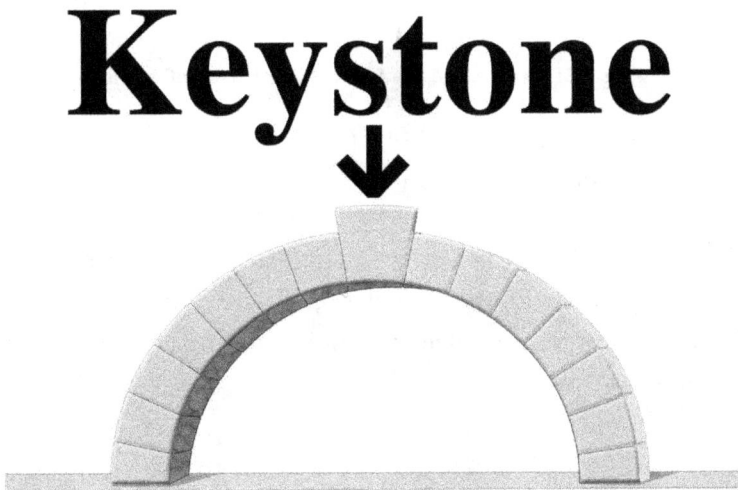

Figure 2-1: Depiction of an arch holding weight with a keystone.

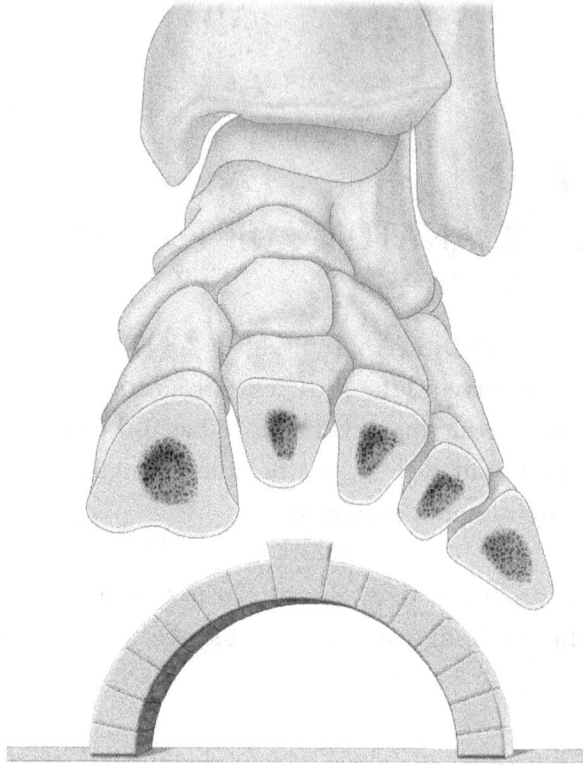

Figure 2-2: The arch of the foot is like an arch of a bridge.

Yet the foot supports the body's weight with a flexibility that can absorb impact.

Unlike a rigid bridge as shown in Figure 2-1, the foot's bones are connected by joints (articulate), allowing for a little bit of flex in the foot to minimize the amount of impact to the knees, hips, and back.

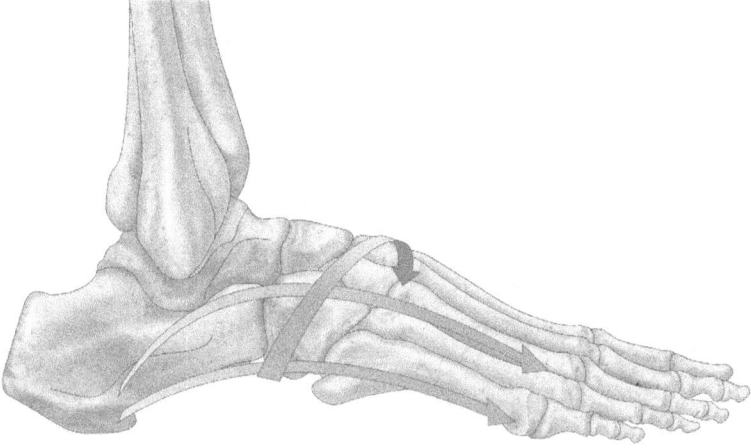

Figure 2-3: Three arches of the foot.

The foot is comprised of not just one, but three arches (as shown in Figures 2-3, 2-4, and 2-5):

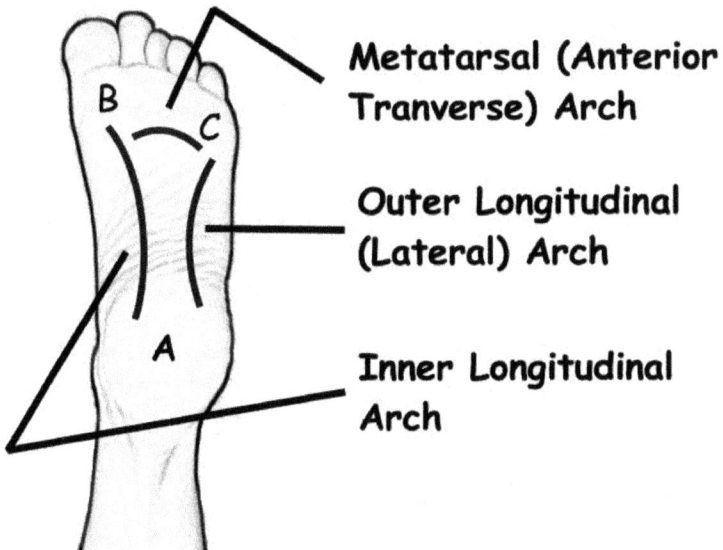

Metatarsal (Anterior Tranverse) Arch

Outer Longitudinal (Lateral) Arch

Inner Longitudinal Arch

Figure 2-4: Three arches of the foot.

1. The inner longitudinal arch (A to B)
2. The traverse (metatarsal) arch (B to C)
3. The outer longitudinal (lateral) arch (A to C)

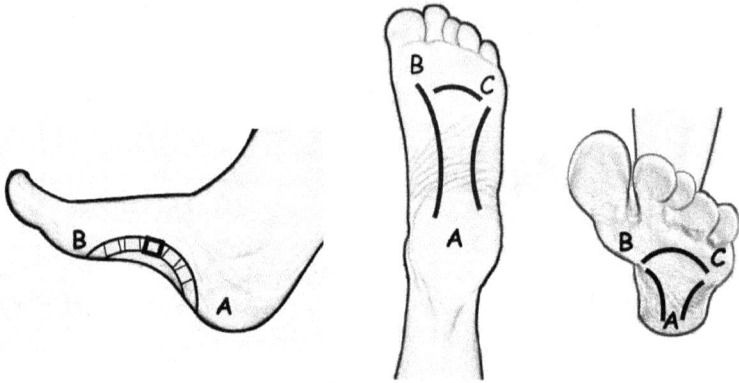

Figure 2-5: The three arches of the foot.

The Bones of the Foot

Unlike the dexterous hand that has eight carpal bones, the weight-bearing foot has seven tarsal bones:

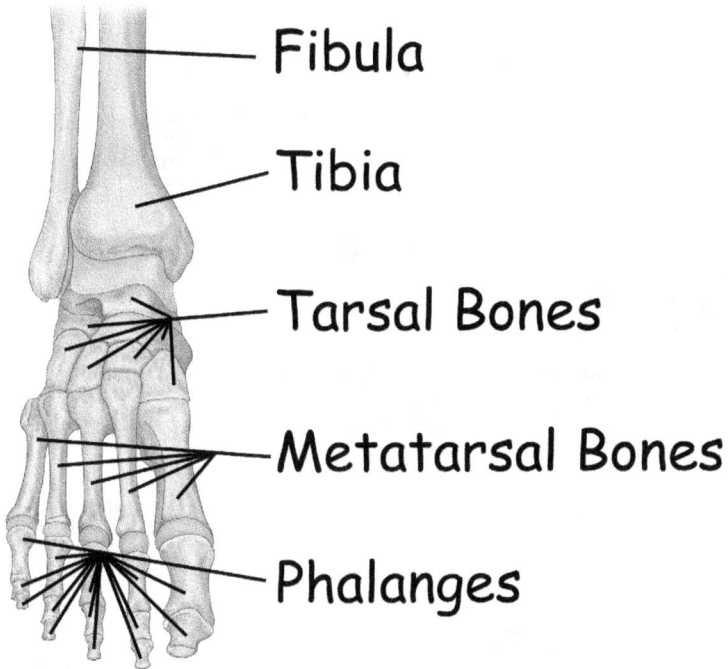

Figure 2-6: Bones of the foot.

The foot has a large bone at the back called the calcaneus that can withstand the heavy burden of supporting the body

The tarsal bones meet up with the metatarsal bones to make the arches of the foot (Figure 2-6). The bones are held in place by ligaments and are moved by the tendons that are attached to the muscles in the lower leg and foot.

The Role of Ligaments

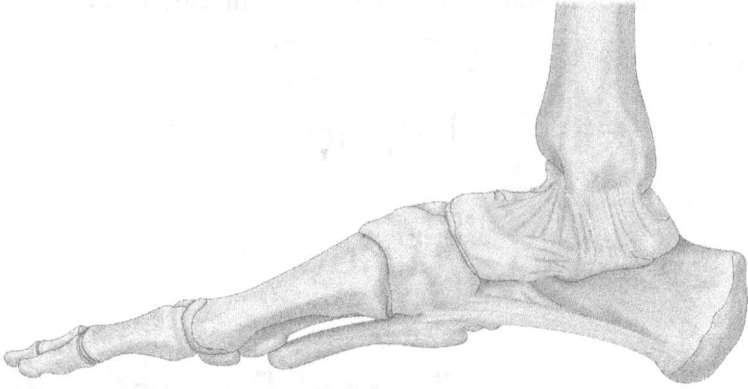

Figure 2-7: Medial ligaments (on the inside) of the foot.

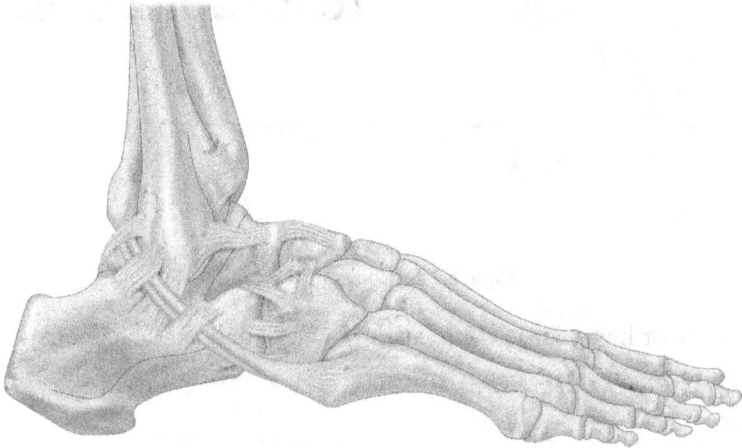

Figure 2-8: Lateral ligaments (on the outside) of the foot.

Ligaments are the strong fibers that hold the weight-bearing bones of your feet in place (Figure 2-7 and 2-8) without having to contract any muscles. Intact, healthy ligaments are imperative to holding up the arches of your feet. Once an arch is flattened, it difficult to regain the height of the arches. Muscles are no help when your arches collapse because muscles are not designed to hold bones in a static position, but to move them. Using orthotics is important when you have collapsed arches because they do some of the work of the ligaments (see Chapter 3 for more details).

When you "roll" your ankle, the ankle bends to such a degree that the ligaments that hold the bones of your foot in place stretch and elongate or tear, becoming weaker. When the ligaments of your ankle and foot are overstretched, the bones can become looser. This is why sprains are so painful; the tissues can get further injured with every step as the bones move outside of their normal position. More on sprains in Chapter 10.

Ankle sprains require stabilization to allow the ligaments to tighten back up as they heal. If the ligaments are not supported during this acute stage, they may heal in an elongated state, and the bones won't have the support they need to function optimally, leading to chronic instability and pain.

Walking Properly

A proper gait cycle involves landing on the calcaneus (heel bone) and picking up the big toe last (Figure 2-9).

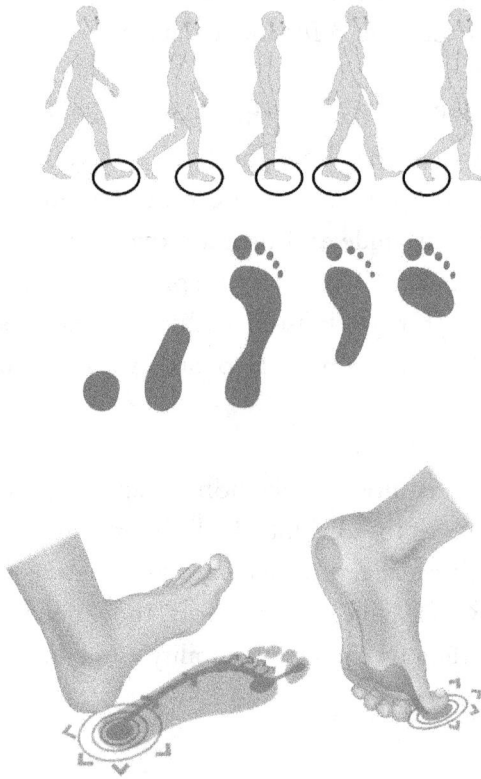

Figure 2-9: Footprint of a healthy gait.

If you have unhealthy feet, they will affect your gait, which can cause pain in your feet, knees, hips, low back, neck, and even shoulders and head.

The following chapters explain how improper foot alignment and function can lead to foot pain and more.

Chapter 3: FOOT PAIN FROM FLAT FEET AND OVERPRONATION

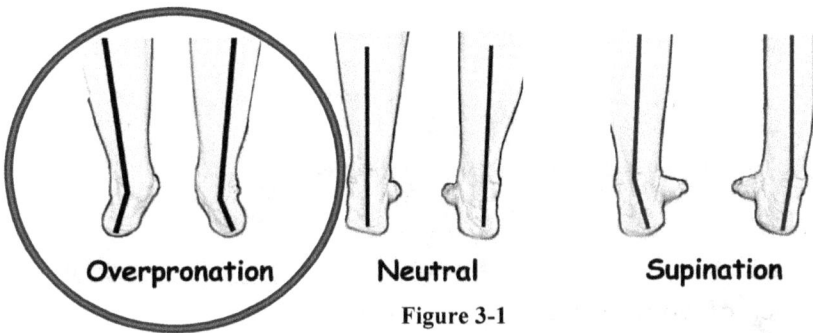

Figure 3-1

THE MOST COMMON CAUSE of foot pain is from collapsing arches, sometimes called flat feet (see Chapter 2 for more about the arches in your feet). The healthy ligaments in your feet hold the tarsal and metatarsal bones firmly in a healthy, biomechanically advantageous arch.

When the ligaments are elongated, whether from overstretching or being stretched repeatedly, they lose their firm hold of the bones, and the arch collapses (Figure 3-2).

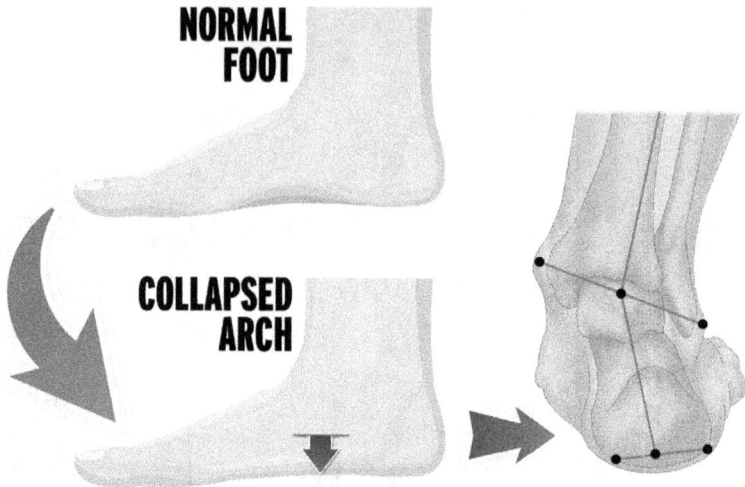

NORMAL FOOT

COLLAPSED ARCH

Figure 3-2: How a collapsed arch affects the ankle.

Collapsed arches are not as good at absorbing the force of impact of your feet hitting the ground. This adds to the compressive force to the foot, causing harm to its tissues.

Not only do collapsed arches increase stress to your feet, but they also strain other areas of the body. When you walk on collapsed arches, the shock waves from your feet landing on the ground during the gait cycle travel up the legs, stressing the knees, hips, and back. Over time, this can lead to pain, not only in the foot, but in other joints as well.

Five Red Flags of Overpronation

Overpronation is when your toes point away from the center of your body. Instead of pointing straight ahead, your feet turn out over seven degrees.

Signs that your feet overpronate include:

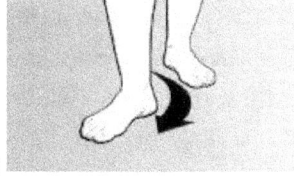

1. Your foot flares while walking:

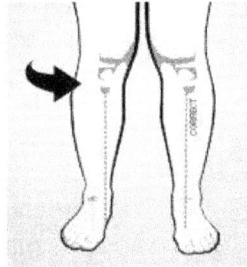

2. Your knees turn in:

3. Your Achilles tendons bow so that your heels point outward:

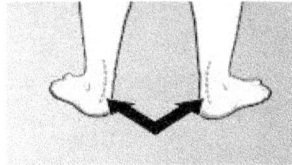

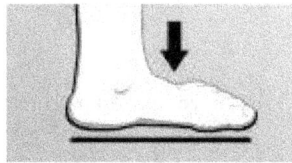

4. Your feet are flat:

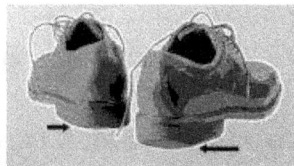

5. Your shoes wear out unevenly:

The Consequences of Overpronation

Oftentimes, a person stresses one foot more than another because they favor one leg. This results in one foot collapsing faster than the other. When this happens, every time a person stands, walks, or does any activity on their feet, the very foundation that they are standing on is imbalanced. It's like walking on a slope that always tilts the pelvis the same way. This causes a greater strain on the hips, pelvis, and back (Figure 3-3).

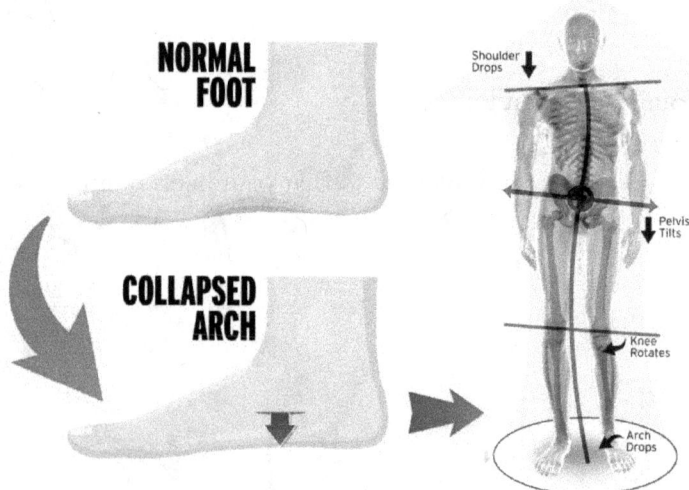

NORMAL FOOT

COLLAPSED ARCH

Shoulder Drops

Pelvis Tilts

Knee Rotates

Arch Drops

Figure 3-3: Unevenly collapsed feet negatively impact other joints of the body.

A collapsed arch affects the gait, causing one foot to overpronate, which is one of the ways the body compensates for the loss of shock absorption.

This is why I am not a fan of minimally supportive shoes. If we were walking on natural surfaces that were soft and uneven, like the types of surfaces our ancestors walked on, then yes, minimalistic shoes would be great. But because we walk on unnatural, hard, flat surfaces, we need arch supports.

Nor am I a fan of shoes with high heels or negative heels. Our bodies were not designed to walk a long distance on a constant uphill or downhill slope.

I have treated women who have worn high heels so often that they developed low back pain; some reached a point that they could not even bring their heels to the ground because their calf muscles were so contracted! It took months of rehabilitation to elongate their calf muscles to the point they could walk in normal shoes without back pain.

More on shoes in Chapter 17.

Using Orthotics

If your arches have collapsed from shoes that lack arch support, this is easily treated with orthotics (Figure 3-4 and 3-5).

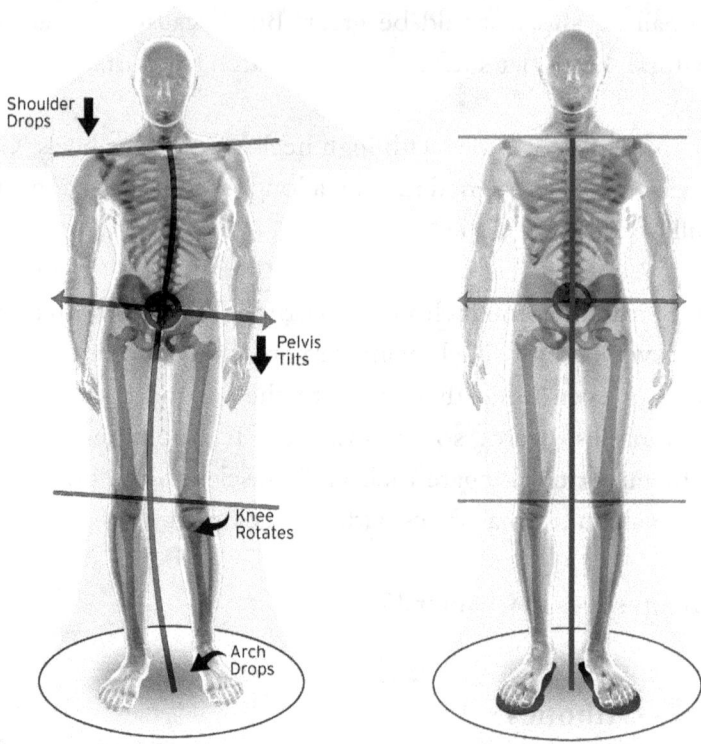

Imbalanced without orthotics

Balanced with orthotics

Shoulder Drops

Pelvis Tilts

Knee Rotates

Arch Drops

Figure 3-4: Orthotics help more than just the feet.

Orthotics are medical devices placed inside shoes to help correct any imbalances in the foot. An example would be custom made insoles (Figure 3-5). Orthotics are not limited custom made insoles, but include heel lifts, ankle supports and more.

Our feet are like race cars. A foot with a healthy arch is like your average rubber tire. It works just fine on any surface.

But when our feet are flat, our bodies don't function as well. When you have a flat tire, you wouldn't replace it with a wooden tire, right? Well, many doctors who treat flat fleet prescribe hard orthotics.

I agree that hard orthotics hold the arches up higher, but they do so at the expense of the foot's function. The foot is designed to collapse a little bit to absorb the impact of landing on the ground. If you have a rigid orthotic, yes, it keeps your arches nice and pretty, but it does not allow the arch to collapse, transferring the shock to your knees, hips, and back.

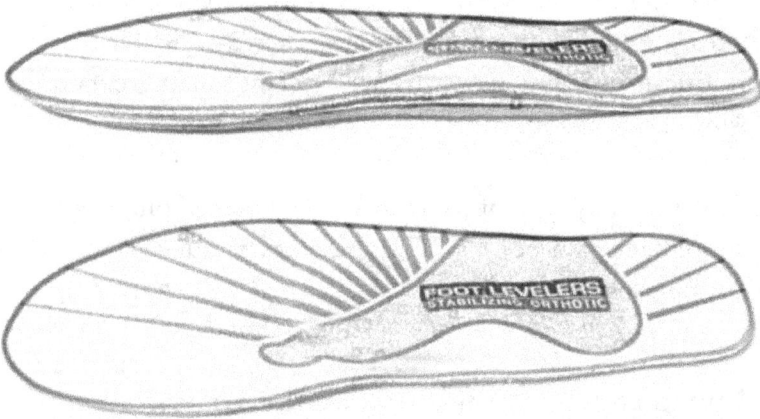

Figure 3-5: Example of orthotics from Foot Levelers™.

I prefer soft orthotics, so I am a big fan of Foot Leveler™ orthotics. They allow for some collapse of the arch while preventing the foot from collapsing to the point of spraining the arch. You want enough support to prevent irritating the tendons and ligaments again and causing pain, but not at the expense of your knees.

If you are morbidly overweight, you may need a rigid orthotic because your weight alone may be enough to crush soft orthotics to the point that they do not provide enough support for your arches.

If your foot pain is severe, you may need the extra support a hard orthotic provides during the healing process because any collapse of the arch (even the normal amount with activity) can re-irritate the tissue as it heals. You should not be doing any high-impact activities at this acute stage, so you do not need the extra cushion of a softer orthotic. A rigid orthotic is a better choice during the acute stage. But once you are well and increasing your amount of physical activity, switch to a soft orthotic to prevent reoccurrences, yet not at the expense of losing shock absorption.

If you have any type of foot pain and are developing knee, hip, and/or back pain, see your chiropractor or podiatrist to discuss your options.

How to Determine if Your Arches Are Collapsing?

To know whether your arches are collapsing, your health provider will examine your feet. They can measure the height of your arch when it is not bearing weight and when it is bearing weight and calculate the difference between the two. A collapse in your arch of more than 3 millimeters is clinically significant. If your arches collapse between 3 and 9 millimeters, orthotics are recommended. If they collapse more than 9 millimeters, then orthotics are required.

Thanks to technology, your healthcare provider can determine the precise height of your arches. You stand on a platform (it looks a little bit like a doctor's scale), and a laser measures the height of your arches and takes a picture of your feet while they are supporting your weight.

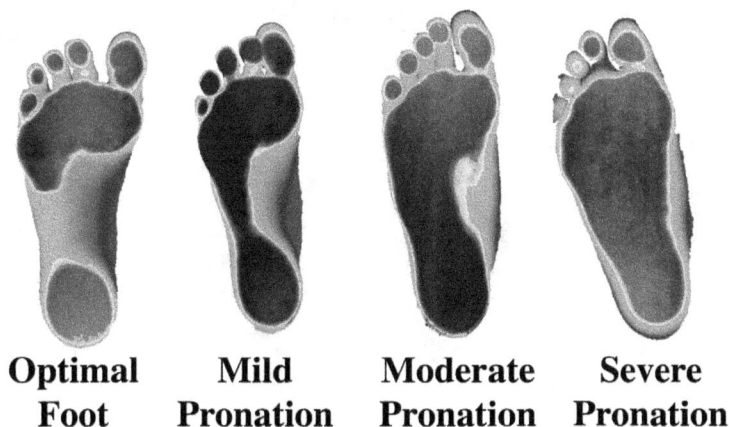

| Optimal Foot | Mild Pronation | Moderate Pronation | Severe Pronation |

Figure 3-6: Scans of different degrees of collapsed feet.

The computer then uses the measurements to produce an image that allows the practitioner to see the degree of arch collapse (Figure 3-6).

The computer color-codes the foot's weight-bearing regions. The regions of the foot that are heavily pressed to the surface are colored red. The areas of the foot that are lightly touching the ground are colored yellow. Tissues off the ground are colored green. Regions of the foot that are high off the ground are colored blue. To see a color example of foot scans, visit www.footlevelers.com.

A healthy weight-bearing foot maintains its three arches, as shown in the first image in Figure 3-6. Collapsed arches will show a broader region of red as the foot flattens on the scanner.

If a scan determines that a pair of orthotics is necessary, more measurements are taken, and the information is sent to a lab to make custom orthotics for your specific needs.

If your pronation is severe, a wedge may be needed to help align your feet and ankles (Figure 3-7).

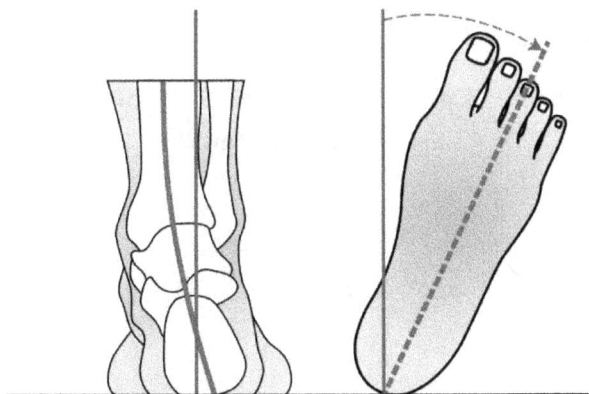

Pronated foot showing incorrect alignment of Achilles Tendon and foot flare.

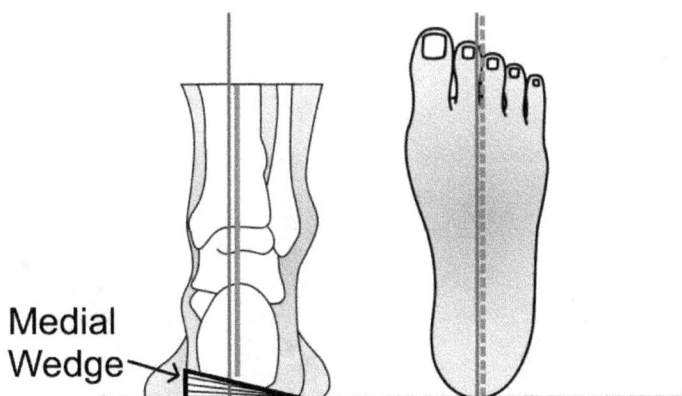

Medial Wedge

Medial placement of SPS wedge corrects misalignment.

Figure 3-7

Basically put, a lot of thought is put into custom-made orthotics. However, the result is less pain and better functioning feet. Better functioning feet reduce strain on your joints, thereby decreasing your risk of needing surgery down the road.

"An ounce of prevention is worth a pound of cure."
—Benjamin Franklin

Chapter 4: SUPINATION

S UPINATION is when the arches of your feet are too high, causing you to walk on the outside of your feet.

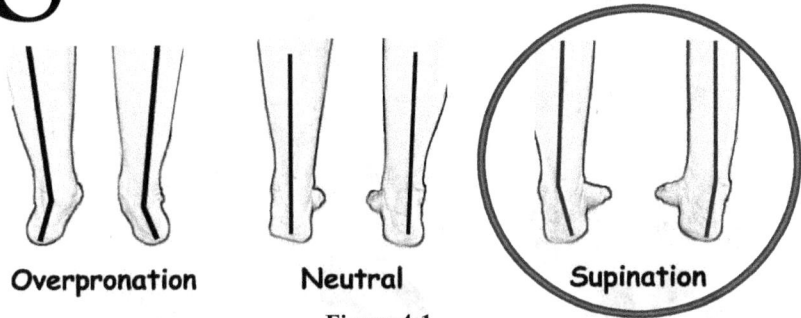

Overpronation   Neutral   Supination

Figure 4-1

The Consequences of Supination

Like overpronation (see Chapter 3), supination affects more than just the feet and ankles. Walking too much on the outside of your feet causes your knees to bow outward. The knees are hinge joints that work best when they bend in a straight position. If you walk with the knees bowed at an angle, the excessive stress of this abnormal motion causes wear and tear over time, leading to degeneration and pain.

Optimal   Supination   Pronation

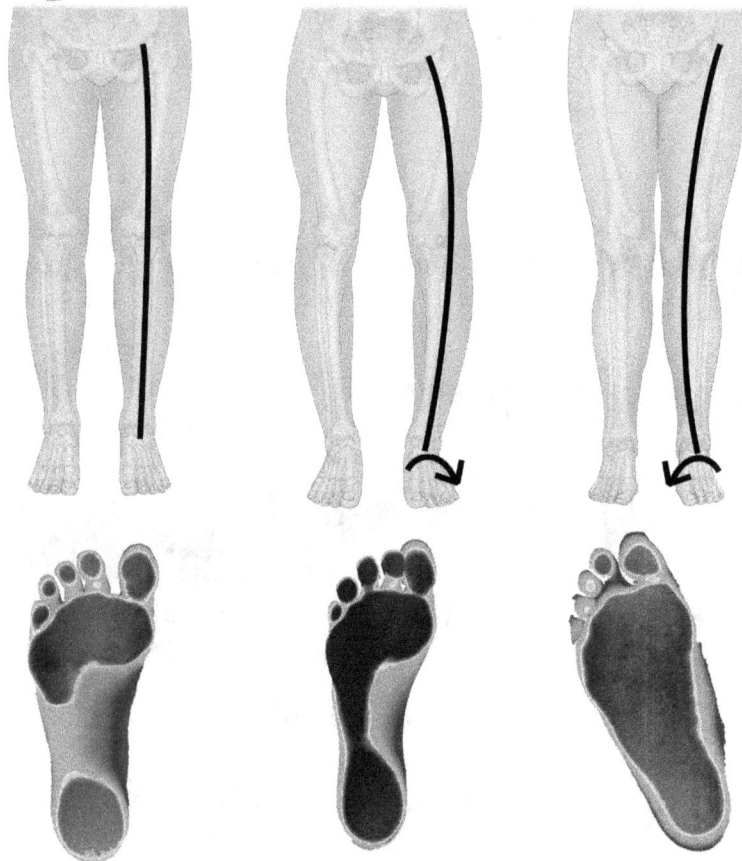

Figure 4-2

Supination of the feet also affects the hips; supination typically causes the legs and hips to overly rotate outward, causing the hips to grind with every step. This extra stress on the hips can lead to early degeneration and pain.

An imbalance of the amount of supination between the left and right foot can cause the pelvis to tilt, straining the back and spraining the sacroiliac joints (the joints in the pelvis).

A foot scan should be performed to determine the degree of supination.

Typically, high arches are more rigid and do not absorb shock as well as a normal arch. Let's go back to the race car analogy. Instead of having regular rubber tires (healthy shock absorbing feet), you have wooden tires (rigid feet). So you need to add more cushion to your feet.

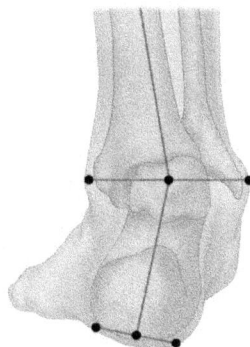

Beware if you just wear soft insoles for the extra cushion; this may cause your arches to collapse over time. I prefer to support high arches with soft, supportive orthotics to provide the cushion that high arches need. Soft orthotics also help prevent high arches from collapsing.

Figure 4-3: Effect of supination on the ankle

Again, I am a big fan of Foot Leveler orthotics, not just for flat feet, but for supination (high arches) as well.

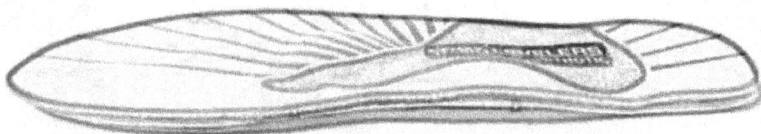

Figure 4-4: Foot Leveler Orthotic

Chapter 5: PLANTAR FASCIITIS

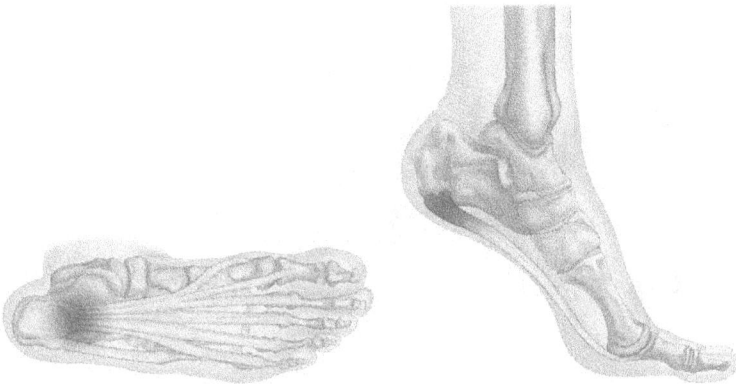

Figure 5-1: The plantar fascia.

COLLAPSED ARCHES strain the plantar fascia (the tissue on the bottom of the foot) more than any other tissue in the feet because the plantar fascia stretches every time the arches collapse. This causes every step to irritate this tissue, which can lead to inflammation and pain.

Plantar fasciitis is inflammation of the plantar fascia. Like any inflamed tissue, it is very tender when moved. It's like having tennis elbow of the foot. However, unlike the elbow, the foot is weight bearing, so just standing irritates the tissue.

To make matters worse, the plantar fascia is the most distal tissue of the body; it is the furthest tissues to supply blood to and drain waste from. Marry this with the fact that the plantar fascia is squished when you bear weight on the foot, and you can understand why this is such a painful condition!

Because we rely on our feet so much, it is difficult to treat and recover from plantar fasciitis.

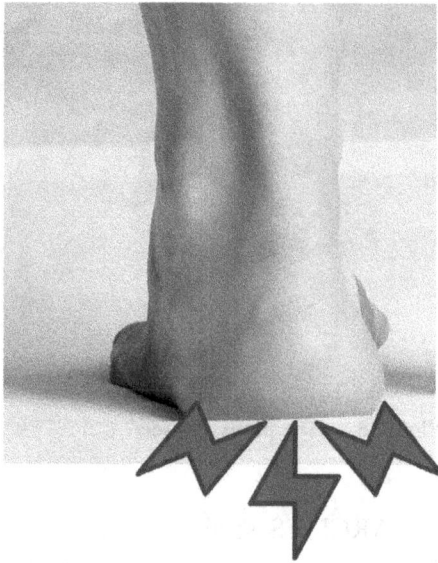

Figure 5-2: Heel pain can be caused by inflamed tissue anchored to it.

Every time your foot hits the ground, the weight of your body compresses the tissues in the heel, squishing out the needed nutrients. Plus, the momentum of the movement causes the arch to strain or sprain. With every step, the ligaments and tendons pull on the bones they are anchored to. This is why people develop more pain with walking (unlike other conditions that are alleviated by walking).

Eventually, walking can inflame the tendons and ligaments to the point that your feet hurt all the time, not just when you walk.

If the foot remains swollen with inflammatory proteins, often the first step is very painful (just like other conditions) and worsens with every step (unlike other conditions).

Treating Plantar Fasciitis

If you suffer from plantar fasciitis, you can recover, but treatment is necessary.

See a healthcare provider to confirm that you have plantar fasciitis. If you do, you need to support the plantar fascia with orthotics. (See Chapter 3 for more about orthotics.)

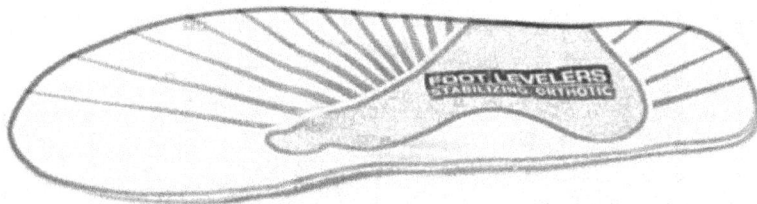

Figure 5-3: Orthotics help plantar fasciitis.

Home care includes heating the calf muscles for five to ten minutes, stretching the lower leg and foot as described in Chapter 19 and then massaging the area of foot that is in pain with ice for two minutes, as described in Chapter 20.

Avoid any activities that cause pain.

Extreme cases may require the use of a boot
to keep the weight off of the plantar fascia.
If you need to wear a boot, make sure to put
an orthotic in it because boots are typically
flat. The lack of arch support can worsen
the plantar fasciitis.

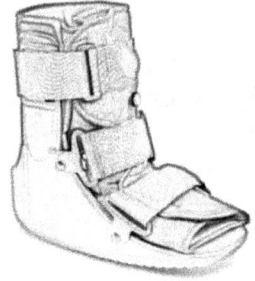

Make sure you find a shoe to wear on your
asymptomatic foot that has a higher sole so your leg lengths
remain the same. You don't want to mess up your back while
trying to heal your plantar fasciitis!

Chapter 6: BUNIONS

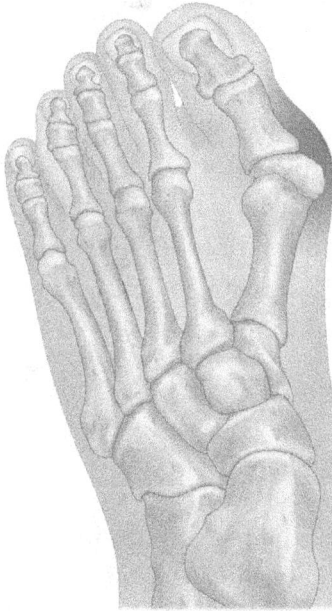

Figure 6-1: Bunion

A BUNION (hallux valgus) develops when the big toe is forced inward from close-toed shoes.

As you toe off when you walk, the big toe bends upward and then presses into the ground to help propel you forward. If the shoes you are wearing are too tight (even just a little), the shoes will press your big toe inward. This compression stresses the joint at the base of the big toe.

Joints under pressure thicken over time to better handle the stressors. When this happens at the base of the big toe, we call it a bunion.

A bunion becomes painful when the stress is enough to cause inflammation.

Oftentimes, the treatment is to put a pin through the joint, immobilizing it so it does not inflame. The problem with this treatment is that it affects how you walk! Because you can't bend your big toe, you have to lift your foot up earlier, which stresses other joints, leading to knee, hip, and/or low back pain.

My suggestion: Try toe spacers.

Toe spacers placed between the first and second toes help the big toe stay in alignment, despite being in close-toed shoes. This prevents the bunion from worsening and may result in decreasing the bunion over time. Bone is not like iron that rusts with time. Bone is living tissue that responds to stressors. Under stress, it thickens. Take the stressor away, and the bone will thin out. It takes years, but better to improve the condition than to have it worsen over time.

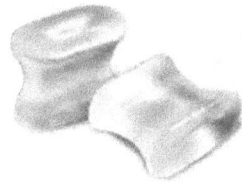

Figure 6-2: Toe Spacers

I wear toe spacers between my big toe and second toe, as well as between my third and fourth toes. The spacers last for more than six months before squishing to a point where they need to be replaced.

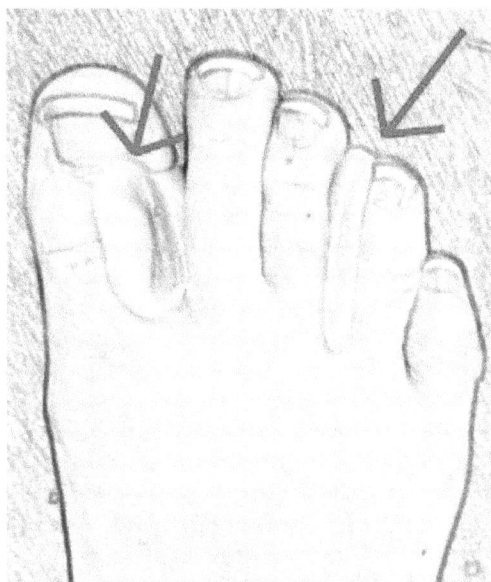

Figure 6-3: Toe spacers (thick for between the big toe and second toe, thin for between the other toes).

I was born with a crooked fourth toe on both feet. My fourth toes curl under my third, creating callouses. This worsened over time, until my mid-thirties, when I started keeping the fourth toes straight with skinny toe spacers that I use when I wear close-toed shoes. That way when I wear sandals, the fourth toe does not curl so deeply under my third toe (like it did in my early thirties). My feet are in better shape in my forties than they were in my thirties!

Here's an interesting fact about spacers. One of my patients was going through toe spacers every few weeks, versus having them last more than six months. Come to find out, she used coconut oil on her feet as lotion. Once she stopped applying the coconut oil on her feet, the toe spacers lasted a lot longer!

If your bunion is moderate to severe, try wearing a bunion splint at night as well. I have saved countless patients from bunion surgery by suggesting they wear a bunion splint at night.

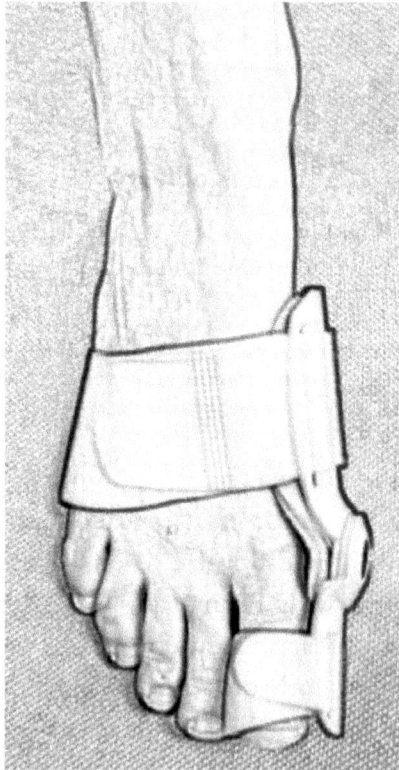

Figure 6-4: A bunion splint.

The foot is designed to walk with the toes straight ahead. Wearing shoes that have narrow toe boxes forces the toe to bend in (hallux valgus). The hinge joint at the base of the big toe enables the toe to bend up and press down as we toe off when we walk.

But if the big toe is forced to bend inward (toward the midline of the body) by a tight-fitting shoe, this abnormal position strains the hinge joint (the first PIP joint). This repetitive strain eventually causes the bones of the joint to thicken and become arthritic. Then a bunion forms.

Again, bones are not like iron that rusts with time. It takes time for them to degenerate and become arthritic, just like it takes time to reverse this process.

To reverse bunions, wear toe spacers to keep the big toe straight during the gait cycle, and wear bunion splints at night to keep the joint neutral as it remodels and heals during sleep.

If something physical causes a musculoskeletal condition, doing the opposite often helps reverse that condition.

Chapter 7: CLAW, MALLET, AND HAMMER TOES

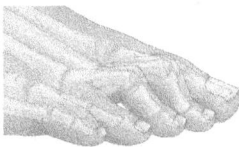 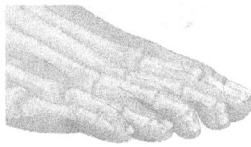 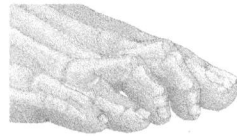

Hammer Toes   **Mallet Toes**   **Claw Toes**

TOES CAN BE A CAUSE of foot pain. Three common problems are hammertoes, mallet toes, and claw toes. These conditions can occur in any of the toes, but typically happen in the three middle toes.

A hammertoe is when the first joint of the toe (the proximal interphalangeal [PIP] joint) bends and is difficult, if not impossible, to straighten (Figure 7-1).

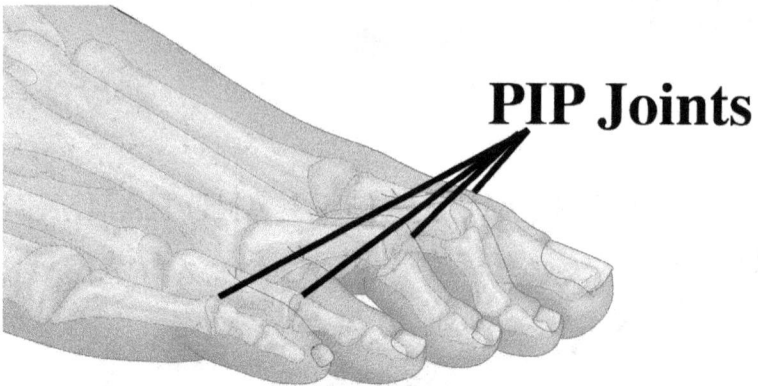

PIP Joints

Figure 7-1: Hammertoes.

Mallet toe occurs when the second joint of the toe (the distal interphalangeal [DIP] joint) bends in this way (Figure 7-2).

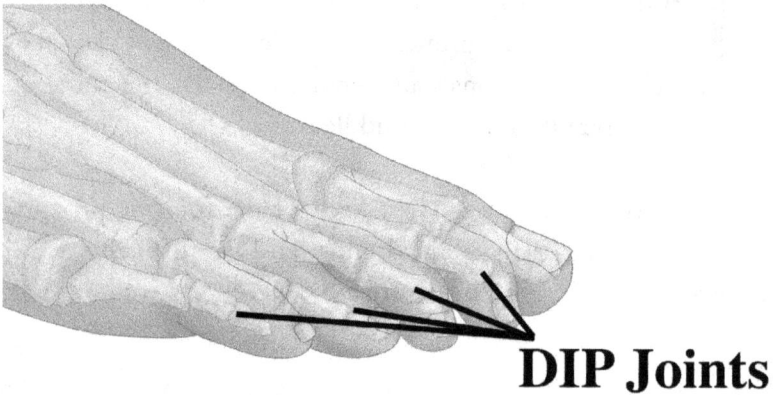

DIP Joints

Figure 7-2: Mallet toes.

A claw toe is when both of the joints bend, and the toe looks like a claw (Figure 7-3).

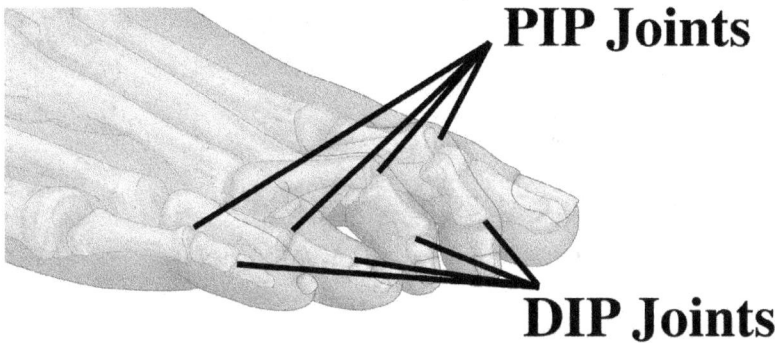

PIP Joints

DIP Joints

Figure 7-3: Claw toes.

These conditions are usually caused by wearing shoes that are too short or too tight. Our feet grow with time, even in adulthood. People often continue wearing the same size shoe they have for years without realizing the harm they are causing their feet. They don't realize their toes are being squished because the toes simply bend to squeeze into the limited space. But over time, this abnormal stress causes the bones to change.

Remember, bones are living tissue that remodel with stress. The good news is if you take the stress away, the bones can remodel to a more normal shape—but this takes years.

Just as with bunions, an ounce of prevention is worth a pound of cure. If you notice your toes are starting to bend in a funny way, you can wear toe tubes to help keep them straight (Figure 7-4). If your shoes are too tight to wear toe tubes, then your shoes are too tight for your feet.

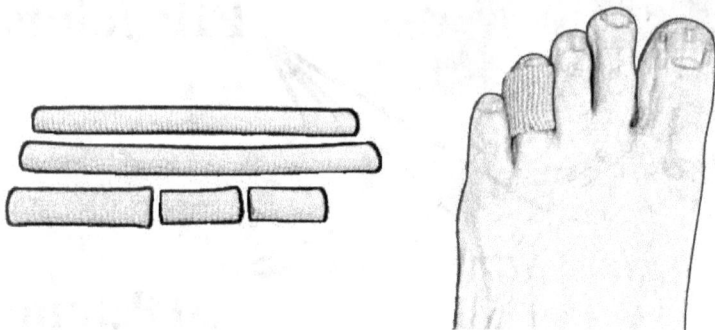

Figure 7-4: Toe tubes.

You can correct hammertoes by holding down your toes with a hammertoe crutch, also known as a hammertoe straighter or hammertoe pad (Figure 7-5)

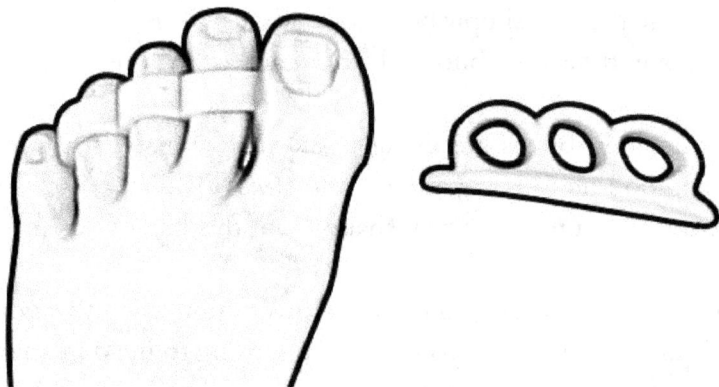

Figure 7-5: Toe pads for bent toes.

These items can be found online or at your local drugstore.

Another cause of bending toes is tightening ligaments or tendons in the foot. Again, this can be from ill-fitting shoes, extremely high arches, injury, diseases or neurological

54

conditions that weaken the muscles of the feet, creating the imbalances that bend your toes.

If your toes are bending abnormally, your healthcare provider should put you through some tests to rule out such diseases and neurologic disorders.

Chapter 8: BONE SPURS

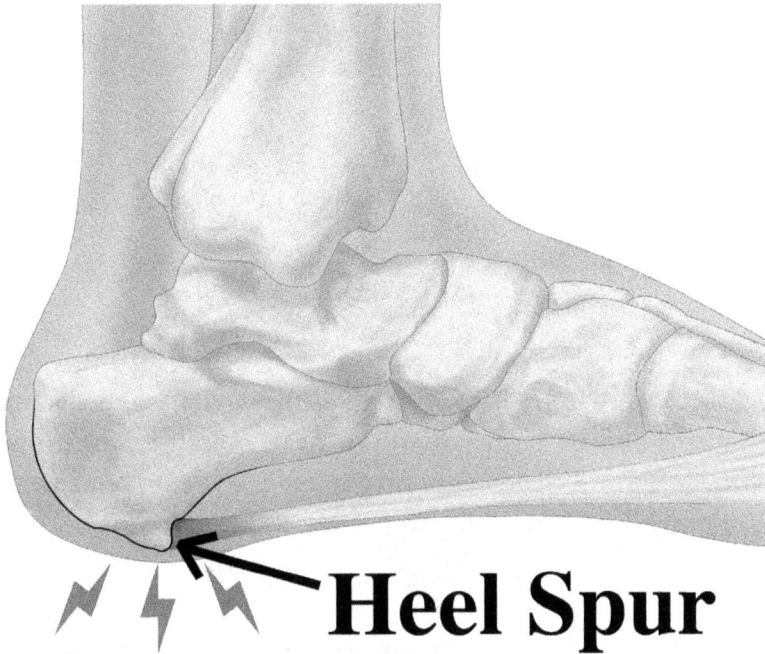

Figure 8-1: A heel spur is an abnormal growth on the bone.

A SPUR DEVELOPS when the heel is under duress, and the bone thickens as a response.

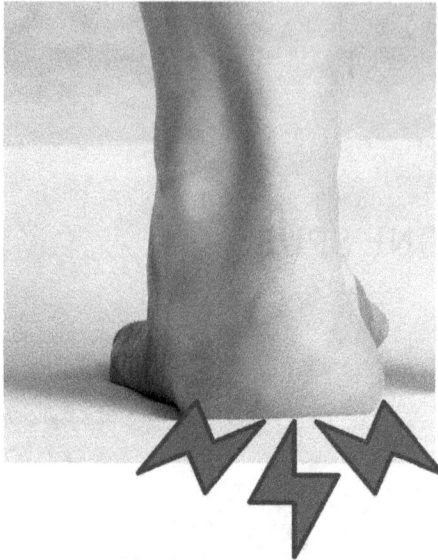

Figure 8-2: Heel pain from a heel spur.

The stress can be due to the arch collapsing, causing the plantar fascia to pull on its insertion on the heel bone. This causes inflammation. Inflammation in a tendon results in bone being laid down, and when this happens in the feet, it causes a heel spur.

The treatment for heel spurs is to use U-shaped silicone heel spur pads (Figure 8-3).

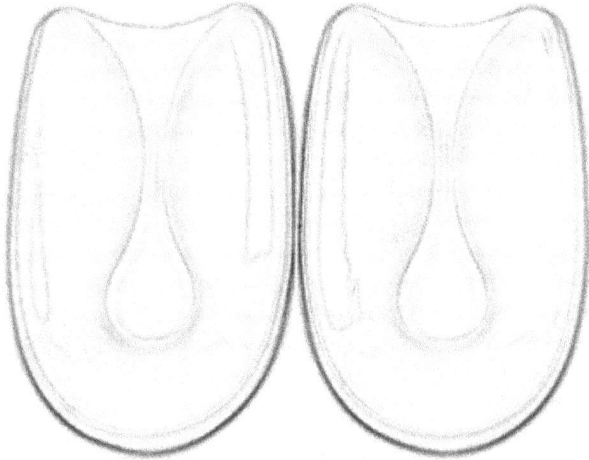

Figure 8-3: U-shaped silicone pads relieve pressure on heel spurs.

Posterior Spur

Spurs can also occur at the top back side of the heel bone from a tight calf muscle. The tight calf muscle causes its tendon, the Achilles tendon, to pull on its insertion at the back of the heel bone (Figure 8-4).

Posterior Heel Spur

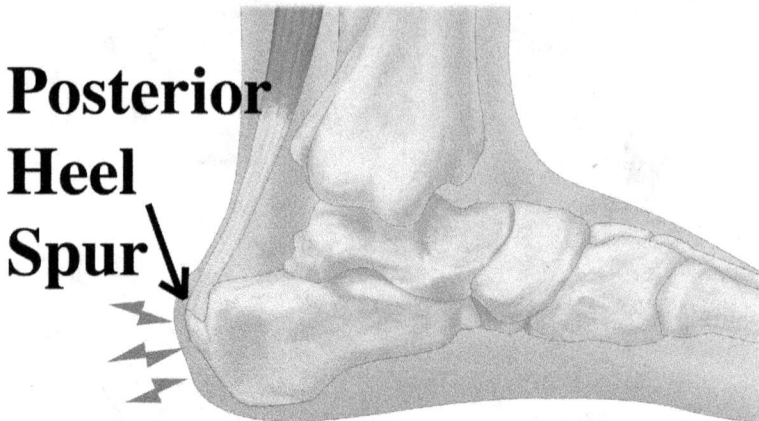

Figure 8-4: Posterior heel spur.

A constant pull on the Achilles tendon can also lead to bursitis, an inflammatory response that can cause bone to be laid down in this region, causing a bone spur on the back of the heel.

The treatment for a posterior heel spur is to heat the calf for 10 minutes, stretch the calf muscle for a few minutes (see Chapter 19 to learn how to stretch the calf muscle), massage the calf muscle (see chapter 20), and then ice the tendon for two minutes. This should be repeated several times a day.

Do not exercise the muscles in the lower legs or feet until the inflammation has calmed down and it no longer hurts to exercise these muscles.

If the heating-stretching-cooling treatment does not work, then you may need to wear an immobilizing boot to take enough pressure off the tendons and bones to allow them to heal, and then work on regaining mobility to the ankle afterward.

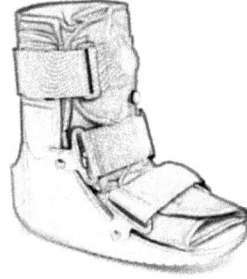

Chapter 9: FOOT PAIN AFTER TRAUMA AND INJURY

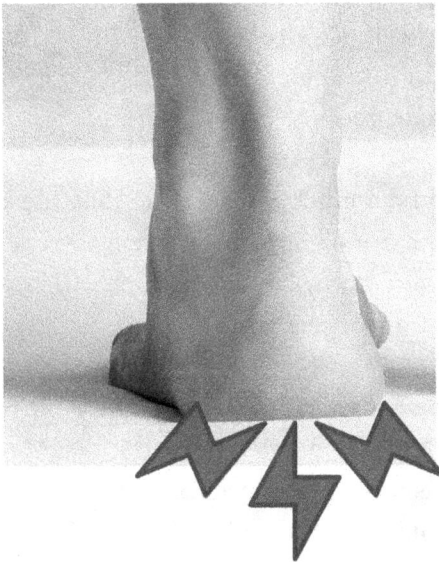

Figure 9-1: Heel pain from injury to the heel bone.

SEVERE FOOT PAIN can be a result of a bone bruise, fracture (hairline, avulsion, or full), or swelling (edema) in a muscle, ligament or bone of the foot. These conditions are usually caused by an injury that involved a strong force (a heavy object landing on the foot; the foot pressing hard against something, like the brake during a car crash; etc.). More on how swelling can cause foot pain in Chapter 14.

Broken Bones

If the force that hit your foot is strong enough to break a bone, the pain is usually so bad that you can't walk more than three steps on the foot. In fact, the three-step test is one of the tests practitioners use to diagnose a broken bone in the foot. If you can't walk more than three steps, a bone is likely broken. The question is, to what degree?

The break may just be a crack in the bone (hairline fracture), or maybe a piece of a bone got torn off (avulsion fracture), or maybe a bone split in two or shattered into three or more pieces (comminuted fracture).

If the bone splits, it is either stable—where the bone maintains its shape and is barely out of place—or not. The line of the fracture may be transverse (straight across the bone) or oblique (where the fracture line is at an angle).

Regardless, a broken bone needs to be braced with either a cast or a boot, or you need to have surgery to set the bone to allow it to heal properly. Your healthcare practitioner will determine which treatment option is best for you.

If you wear a boot or a cast, make sure the other foot has footwear with a high or tall insole to minimize the imbalance of wearing a boot on one leg and not the other. If you don't, your knee and hip will be higher on the side wearing the boot than the knee and hip on the other side, which can cause knee, low back, neck, and head pain (just like a leg length inequality can). To learn more, check out my *Combat Neck Pain* and *Combat Low Back Pain* books.

If you have to wear a cast, make sure the doctor sets your foot with your arch in neutral. I have treated too many patients who have had a flat foot after wearing a cast without arch support for a few weeks. The flat cast flattened their arch! If you have an air cast boot, you can put an arch support in it to support your arches while your bones heal.

After your bone has healed, you need to have physical therapy and chiropractic manipulation to restore the range of motion to your foot and ankle. Remember, if you don't use it (in this case, you're the muscles and joints of the ankles), you lose it. After being immobilized in a cast or boot, your ankle stiffens and your lower legs muscles weaken from not moving for weeks. So, you have to work on restoring the range of motion in your foot and ankle with chiropractic treatment and re-strengthen your foot and lower leg muscles with physical therapy.

You may also need to have your spine adjusted after straining your back from walking with a heavy cast or boot on one side for so long.

Bone Bruise

A bone bruise happens when a force causes a tear in a blood vessel inside the bone. Bone is a hard structure with sensitive nerves. When blood leaks into the bone, it has no where to go and causes pressure on the structure inside the bone. Nerves scream with pain under this pressure.

I have found that if a patient cannot bear weight for more than three steps, yet X-rays and CT scans fail to find a fracture, but bruising or swelling is apparent, then treating the injury like a fracture for a few weeks is best.

I had a patient who had swelling in her tarsal bone, but would not wear her boot. The boot was awkward and she didn't have a fracture, so she was convinced it was not worth the hassle to wear the boot. She preferred to wear an ankle brace; it provided enough pain relief while wearing it, but her injury wasn't getting any better. A steroid injection gave her relief for ten days, but then the pain came back. When she was told that she would need surgery, she finally decided to be more committed to using the boot. She wore it faithfully, and within two weeks, the pain subsided.

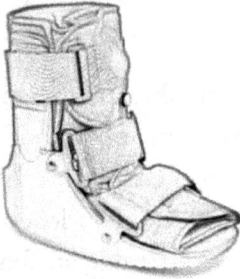

Special Note on Foot Pain in Children

If a child has foot or ankle pain after an injury, it is imperative to check if it has affected the growth plate, either directly by a fracture or indirectly through the blood supply to the growth plate.

If the growth plate gets damaged while it is still growing, the damage will affect the growth of that bone, forever affecting the function of the joints above and below it (Figure 9-2).

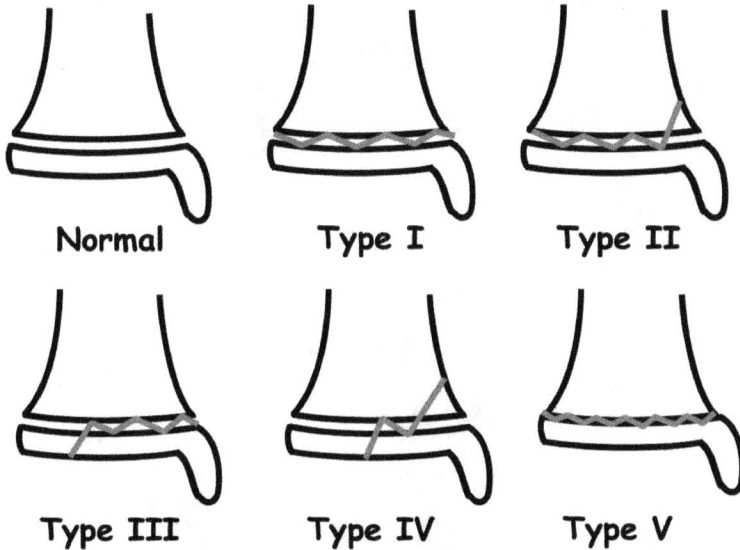

Figure 9-2: Depicting the different ways a bone can fracture at a growth plate.

A Salter-Harris fracture is an especially serious break of a growth plate. This fracture occurs at the end of the tibia (the larger of the two bones in the lower leg) and can affect the length of this weight-bearing bone. If the tibia stops growing, that leg will be shorter than the other.

You do not want to ignore or undertreat this injury.

Having one leg shorter than the other will cause a lifelong foundational imbalance that can lead to chronic knee, hip, low back, and neck pain and headaches.

If a child has a Salter-Harris fracture, the child needs to be seen by an orthopedic surgeon who specializes in children to determine the best treatment option for their specific injury.

Chapter 10: SPRAINS and STRAINS

Signs/Symptoms	Grade I	Grade II	Grade III
Tendon	No tear	Partial tear	Complete tear
Loss of function	Minimal	Some	Great
Pain and swelling	Minimal	Moderate	Severe
Bruising	None (or minimal)	Yes	Severe discoloration
Able to bear weight	Yes	With some difficulty	With great difficulty or cannot

IF YOU HAVE ROLLED your ankle, you likely sprained your ankle ligaments and/or strained the muscles of your ankle. The question is, to what degree? If the area has minimal swelling and you can walk with minimal pain, then you likely have a mild to moderate sprain (grade I or II).

The treatment for a grade I or II sprain is RICE, which stands for:

- Rest
- Ice
- Compression
- Elevation

If you have a grade III strain, there is some debate on the treatment. If you are a professional athlete and don't have time to allow conservative treatments to work, surgery is often the treatment of choice. But if you have the time to allow your body to heal, try conservative approaches first (bracing and RICE, followed by physical therapy, chiropractic manipulation, massage, etc.). If that fails, then you may consider surgery.

Another way to sprain or strain your foot is during a motor vehicle collision. Even a minor impact can sprain the ligaments and strain the muscles of the foot and lower leg, especially if you brace for impact or slam on the brakes (Figure 10-1).

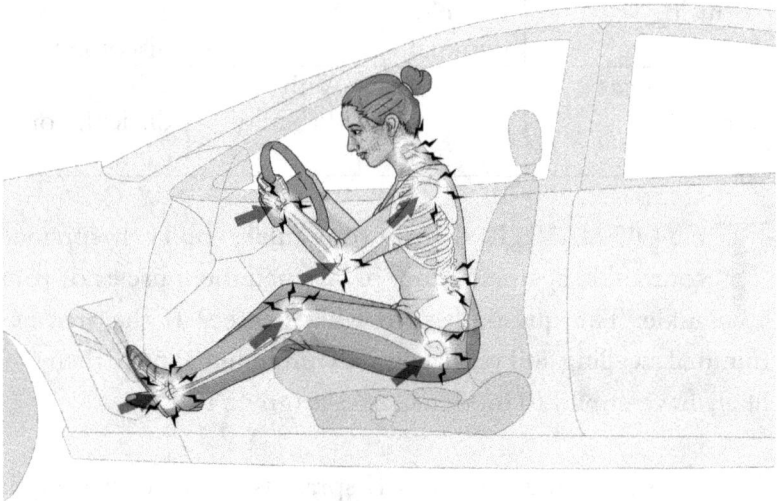

Figure 10-1: A motor vehicle collision can injure the foot.

To learn more about how car crashes can affect the body, check out my book, *Whiplash to Wellness: A Chiropractor's Journey.*

Chapter 11: FOOT PAIN CAUSED BY THE SCIATIC NERVE

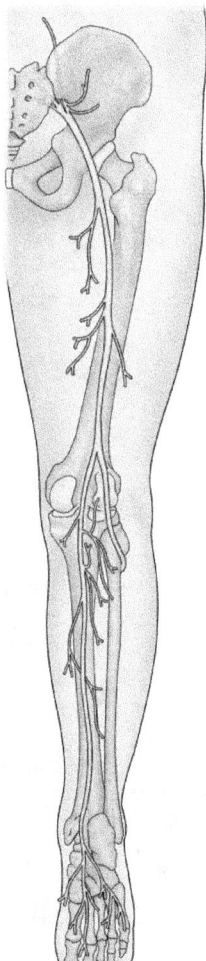

Figure 11-1: Sciatic nerve.

T HE NERVE that transmits signals to and from the foot is the sciatic nerve (Figure 11-1). If something is wrong with the foot, the sciatic nerve transmits the sensation of pain to the brain. But if the top of sciatic nerve is pinched, it causes the sensation of leg pain all the way to the foot (Figure 11-2).

I have seen cases of low back and sacroiliac conditions express as foot pain without the leg pain.

If your foot pain is due to a pinched nerve in your low back, check out my book *Combat Low Back Pain* to learn more about how to get your back well so it no longer causes pain in your foot.

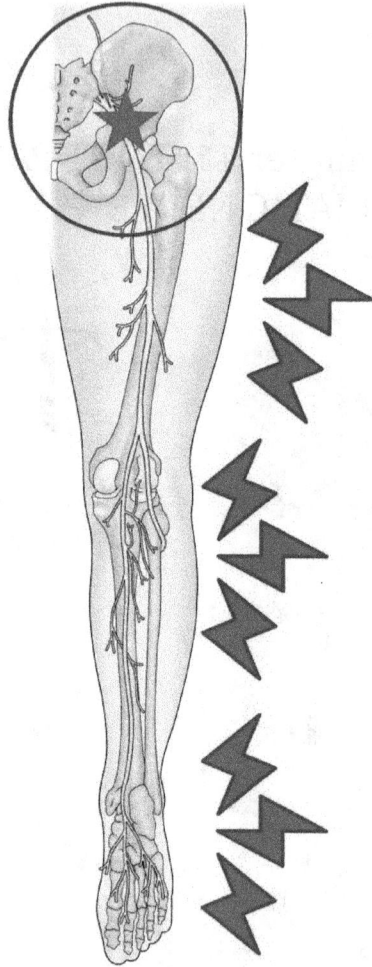

Figure 11-2: A "pinched" sciatic nerve causes the sensation of pain running down the leg to the foot.

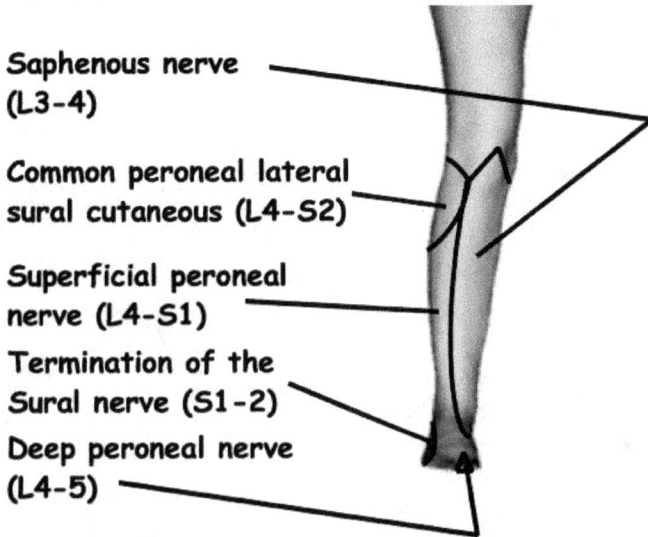

Saphenous nerve
(L3-4)

Common peroneal lateral
sural cutaneous (L4-S2)

Superficial peroneal
nerve (L4-S1)

Termination of the
Sural nerve (S1-2)

Deep peroneal nerve
(L4-5)

Figure 11-3: This image shows the regions of the lower leg that the different branches of the sciatic nerve supply.

Branches of the sciatic nerve can be squished by muscles in the lower leg. When this happens, you usually feel pain at the site of the muscle as well as pain that radiates to the region in the leg that the nerve supplies (Figure 11-3).

For example, if the peroneus muscle on the lateral (outer) side of the leg is tight, it can put pressure on the superficial peroneal nerve, causing pain in the lateral side of the low leg (Figure 11-4). It can also put pressure on the deep peroneal nerve, causing pain between the first and second toes.

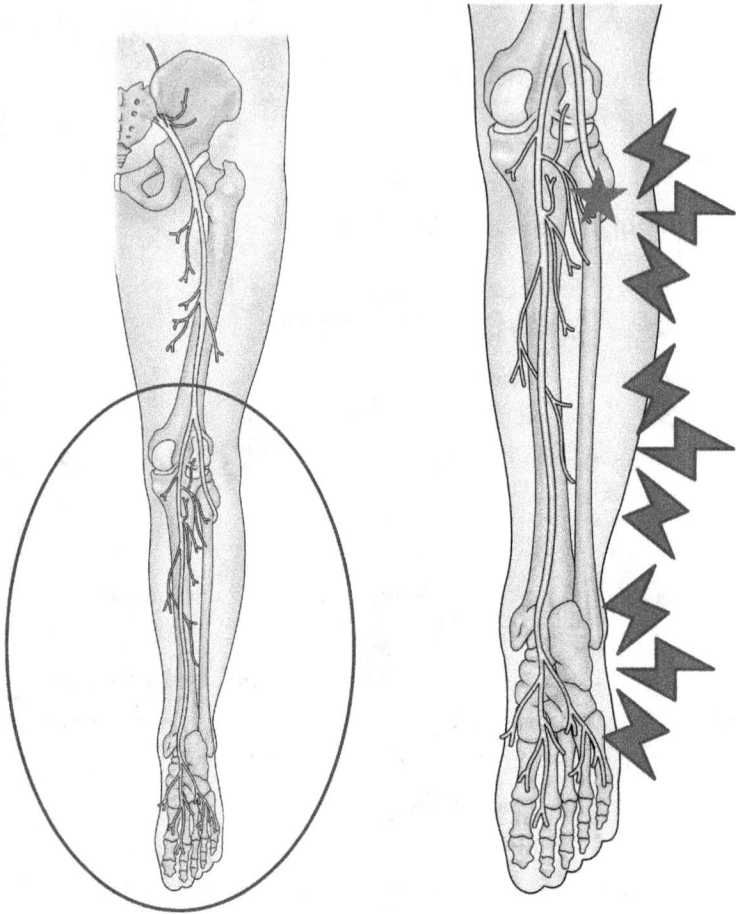

Figure 11-4: Sciatic nerve pinched at the knee causing leg and foot pain.

A tight peroneus muscle can cause foot pain (Figure 11-5), but if the compression is deep and intense enough, it can interrupt the nerve's ability to make a muscle contract. When this occurs, the foot drops (the medical term being "foot drop"). If you notice your ability to raise your toes and foot is weakening, the nerve needs to be immediately decompressed, which may require surgery.

Stretching your calf muscles as in Chapter 19 and massaging your peroneus muscle as in Chapter 20 should alleviate the pain. If it does not resolve or worsens in any way, talk with your healthcare provider. Sometimes surgery is needed to decompress the nerve at this level. If you wait too long, your nerve can be permanently damaged from being under too much pressure for too long.

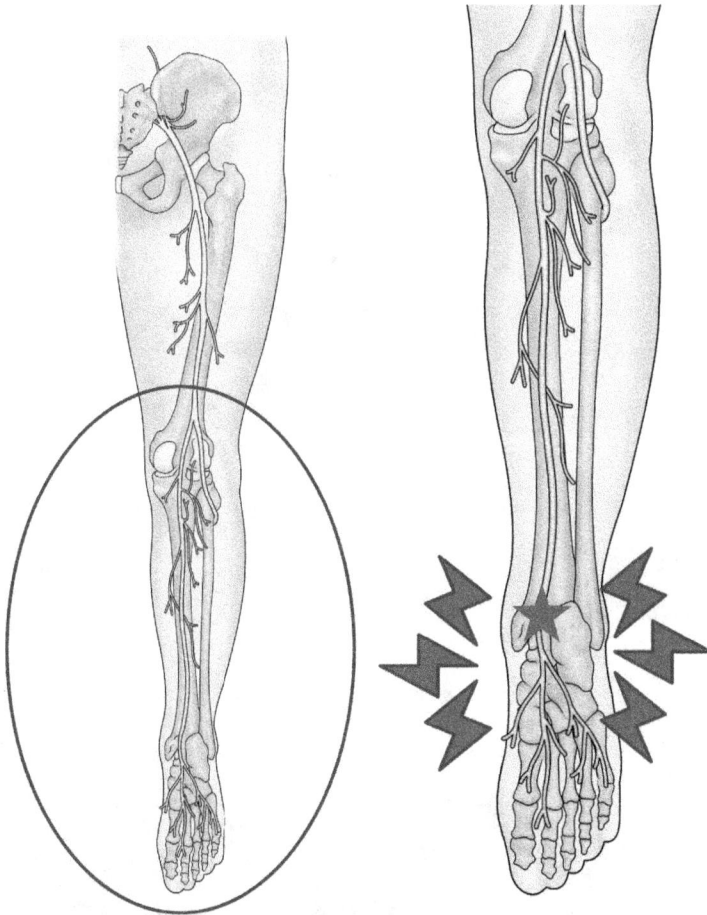

Figure 11-5: Pinched branch of the sciatic nerve causing foot pain.

If the irritation of the nerve is at the ankle, you will feel pain in the foot. Tarsal tunnel syndrome is where a branch of the sciatic nerve is pinched at the ankle. If it is pinched here, try stretching the calf and foot as in Chapter 19. If it does not resolve, again, talk to your healthcare provider to see if decompressive surgery is required.

Chapter 12: MORTON'S NEUROMA

MORTON'S NEUROMA is a condition in which swollen tissues place pressure on a nerve between the metatarsals of the foot or the nerve itself is thickened. The inflammation makes it very painful to bear weight, wear shoes, or walk. Oftentimes patients with Morton's neuroma find that wearing close-toed shoes is almost unbearable and wearing sandals is much more comfortable.

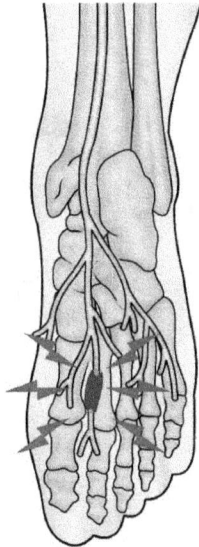

Figure 12-1: Morton's neuroma.

Morton's neuroma is usually caused by wearing shoes that are too tight at the front of the foot, causing the bones and the tissues between the bones of the foot to rub the nerve raw. This causes the tissues between the bones to swell and illicit even more pain. The pain worsens with walking.

You can lessen the pain by stretching the bones of the foot apart. Spreading the bones apart allows more space for the lymph to drain, increases blood flow (which brings nutrients in and waste out), and takes pressure off the nerves, allowing them to heal.

Treatment involves massage (Chapter 20) stretches (Chapter 19) toe spacers, metatarsal pads to cushion the forefoot (Figures 12-2 and 12-3), minimizing weight-bearing activities, ice, and topical anti-inflammatories (like Cryoderm and other topicals mentioned in Chapter 22)..

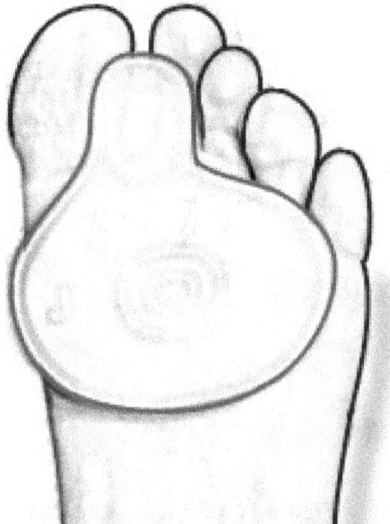

Figure 12-2: Metatarsal gel pads can be worn to reduce pressure on the nerve, allowing it to calm down and heal.

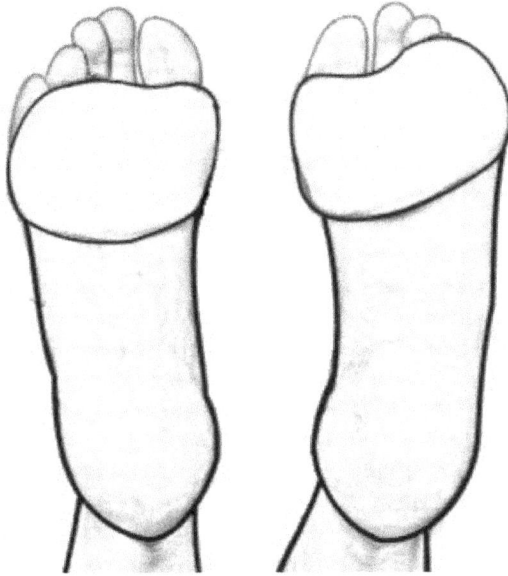

Figure 12-3: Forefoot foam pads can be worn to reduce pressure on the nerve, allowing it to calm down and heal.

If these do not work, talk to your health care provider about orthotics, injections, and surgery as possible treatment options for Morton's neuroma.

Chapter 13: PLANTAR WARTS, CALLUSES, AND ATHLETE'S FOOT

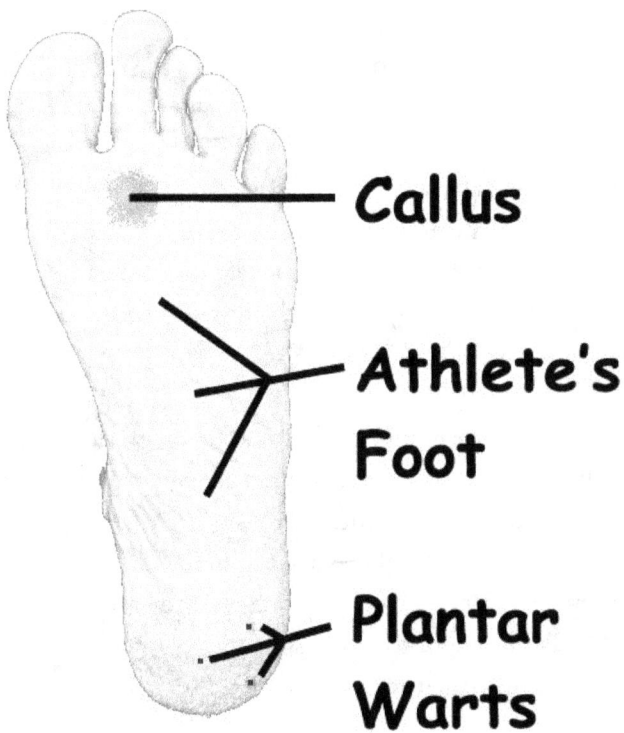

Figure 13-1: Topical foot conditions that can cause foot pain.

FOOT PAIN can be caused by surface conditions on the skin or just below the skin (Figure 13-1), not just musculoskeletal conditions.

Plantar Wart

If you have focal foot pain with walking, check for a grainy growth on the sole of your foot. The pain may be from walking on a plantar wart. Plantar warts are typically found on the bottom (the plantar aspect) of your foot. Hence, the name plantar warts.

Warts are caused by a virus. We are all exposed to such viruses, but a healthy immune system fights them off. Most people who develop warts do so during a time of stress, during which their immune system is compromised, allowing the virus to flourish and warts to develop.

If your pain is from a wart, the wart will often go away on its own. I believe the more attention you give the wart, the more it grows. Countless patients have sworn that putting a small piece of duct tape on the wart for a few weeks until it goes away gets rid of the wart. They believe they are suffocating the wart. I believe it works because they believe it will work and gets their mind off of it.

Warts are a sign of stress. Stress weakens the immune system, allowing the virus to flourish. Then the wart becomes a stressor itself.

The triad of wellness—sleep well, eat well, and move well—is the answer.

Callus

Another possible cause of a focal pain in the foot is a callus. A callus is a thickening of the skin in response to extra pressure. Just like our bones, skin also thickens in response to extra stress.

The formation of a callus can a sign of improper foot biomechanics, and orthotics may be necessary. Wearing orthotics takes the pressure away so the skin stops thickening in that area.

A callus doesn't hurt on its own, but if it is hard and large enough, it may exert enough pressure on the foot tissue to cause pain (like a pebble would in your shoe).

You can remove a callus by soaking your feet in warm water for 10–20 minutes, scrubbing it off with a pumice stone, and applying moisturizer on the region of the callus daily. You can also go to a pedicurist to have the callus professionally removed with a pedicure.

Severe cases may require a podiatrist to burn them off or surgically remove them. A podiatrist may also address the foot condition that is causing the callus to form.

Athlete's foot

Another condition that can irritate your feet is athlete's foot (a fungal infection), but this typically is itchy, not painful. Fungus likes to grow in dark, moist regions, and if your feet are often sweaty, it is a prime location for fungal growth. Keeping your feet dry and clean helps prevent athlete's foot. Applying antifungal creams and powders may also be warranted.

If you have any cause to believe your foot pain is due to a topical condition, seek the advice of a dermatologist.

Chapter 14: PROLONGED SITTING AND THE EFFECT ON YOUR FEET

WHILE YOU'RE SITTING, your hips are bent, and the hip flexor muscles are in a contracted and shortened state. This impairs the lymphatic and venous drainage out of your legs, increasing your risk of varicose veins.

Veins are the blood vessels that return blood to the heart. The pressure is lower in veins than arteries, so valves in these vessels prevent any backflow away from the heart. Veins also rely on the skeletal muscles surrounding them to contract and relax to help pump the blood along.

These valves weaken with stressors like not moving enough (standing or sitting too long), excess pressure from being overweight, injury, genetic weakness, or from poor diet limiting their repair. If the valves are weak, blood can flow in the wrong direction, engorging the section of vein ahead of a valve, resulting in what we call varicose veins.

Sitting and DVT

Worse, excessive sitting increases your risk of developing deep vein thrombosis (DVT). DVT is a potentially fatal condition where a blood clot forms in a vein, breaks off, travels through the circulatory system and gets stuck in the lungs. There the clot, now called a pulmonary embolism, blocks the blood supply to the lungs, which can be fatal without medical treatment.

Sitting and Foot Pain

At a minimum, prolonged sitting increases swelling of the legs, and over time, the swelling can become uncomfortable and even painful.

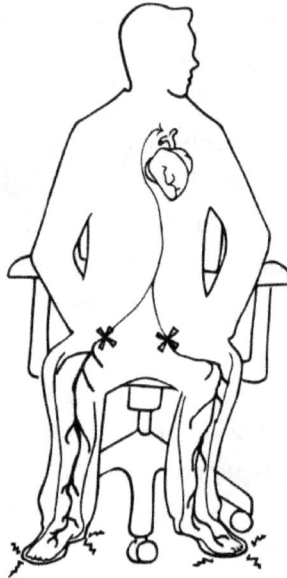

Figure 14-1: Prolonged sitting can cause foot pain.

I have had patients come to me thinking they have plantar fasciitis because they feel severe foot pain when they first stand up. Upon questioning, I discover that their pain improves with walking. This tells me they don't have plantar fasciitis, but likely are experiencing pain caused by swollen lower extremities.

When your feet are swollen, it hurts to bear weight at first. As you move around, the fluids causing the swelling drain, and the pain lessens. It doesn't take a noticeable amount of swelling to be painful. Patients who have swelling caused by too much sitting are often relieved to find out they don't need to buy expensive orthotics.

Other Causes of Swollen Feet

Feet can also swell from standing for long periods of time on a regular basis, flying in airplanes, long commutes (sitting too long without moving), genetic weakness of the valves of the blood and lymph vessels that allows backflow of fluid, or damaged vessels.

Backflow in the veins and/or lymph vessels puts even more pressure on valves and causes them to stretch apart, allowing even more back flow. Like a balloon, once the valves have been stretched, it's easier for them to stretch again, making the valves less able to hold back further backflow.

To relieve pain from weak valves, you can perform the Foot ABCs for Lymphatic Drainage (described in Chapter 19) and elevate your feet often. This drains the lower extremities of the excess fluid.

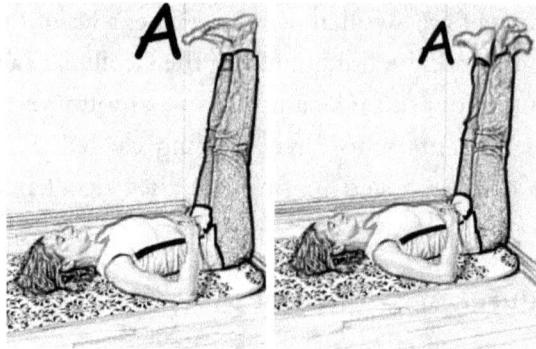

Figure 14-2: Lymphatic drainage.

If the valves are damaged enough, the relief will be temporary because standing up will cause the legs to swell again.

If raising the feet above the heart is not enough to provide lasting relief, you may need to wear compression stockings. You can choose from a variety of compression hose that come in different lengths and amounts of pressure.

Graduated compression socks are effective at preventing and treating varicose veins and swelling of the lower extremities. They gently squeeze the vein and lymph vessel walls together so they can close and prevent the backflow from occurring.

Usually medical compression stockings are 15 mmHg or higher to compress the legs enough to support the veins and lymph vessels of the lower legs.

On long work days, I personally use CopperJoint Performance Compression Socks (Figure 14-3).

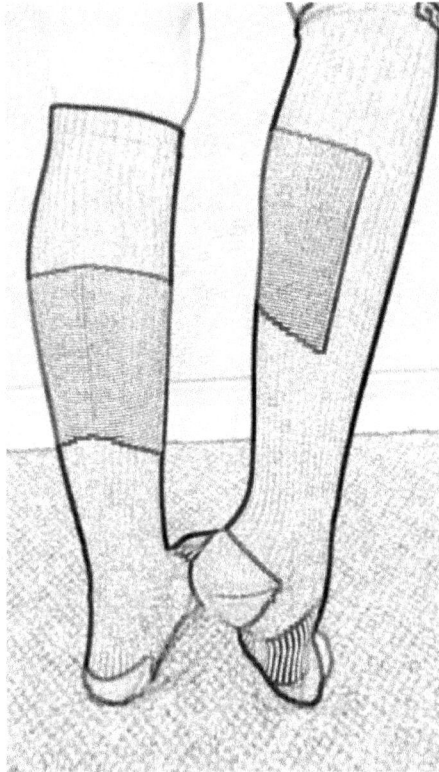

Figure 14-3: My CopperJoint Performance Compression Socks

To learn more about them, check them out on Amazon.com.

Chapter 15: FOOT PAIN FROM CRAMPS

CRAMPS ARE OFTEN the result of dehydration and mineral deficiencies. Such deficiencies include, but are not limited to, calcium, magnesium, and potassium. If people suffer from night cramps, I suggest they take a pill with calcium, magnesium, vitamin D, and a mineral blend before going to sleep. In addition to alleviating cramps, taking such a blend helps you sleep at night. I also suggest they take the pill with a full glass of water (if not two), especially if they are not good about drinking water throughout the day.

Drink Plenty of Water

All tissues in our body need water. Dehydration affects blood pressure, muscle tension, and joint and fascia lubrication, all of which can lead to muscle cramps. (Fascia is the lining that covers muscles and organs in your body, separating the different tissues while holding everything together.)

You can calculate how much water you need to drink by multiplying your body weight by 2/3 (0.66). The result is the number of ounces of water you should drink in a day. For example, I weigh about 125 pounds, so I should drink approximately 83 ounces a day (125 x 2/3 = 82.5). Now, for every half hour you exercise, you should add at least 11 ounces. This is why I try to drink at least 96 ounces (three 32-ounce containers) of water a day.

If you drink black tea, coffee, and/or alcohol, you need to drink even more water. These beverages dehydrate you because they tamper with your anti-diuretic hormone (ADH).

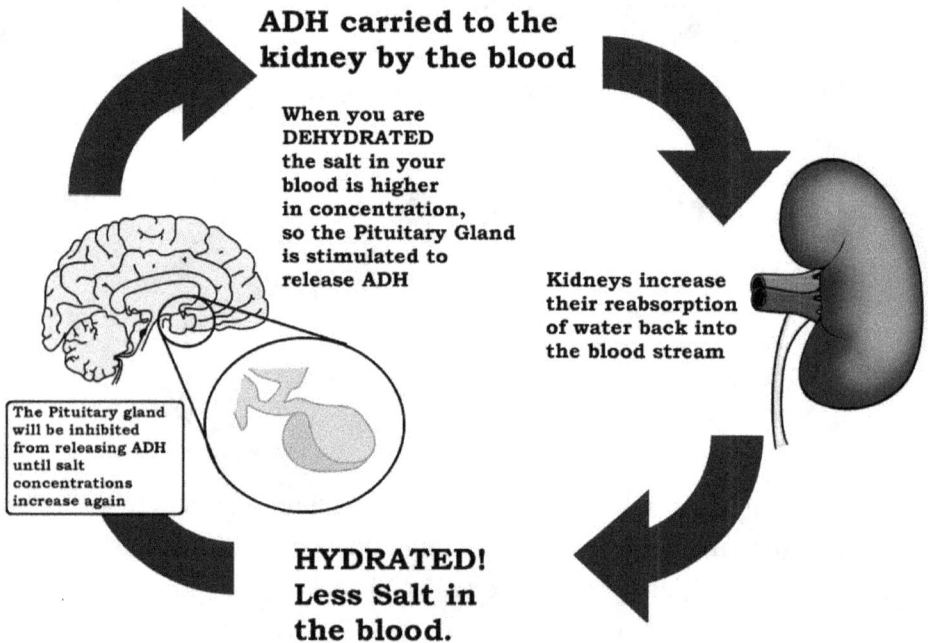

ADH carried to the kidney by the blood

When you are DEHYDRATED the salt in your blood is higher in concentration, so the Pituitary Gland is stimulated to release ADH

Kidneys increase their reabsorption of water back into the blood stream

The Pituitary gland will be inhibited from releasing ADH until salt concentrations increase again

HYDRATED! Less Salt in the blood.

Figure 15-1: How the body regulates water.

The hypothalamus (a part of your brain) detects how much water is in the blood. If the water content is low, the blood has a higher salt content. The pituitary gland (your body's master gland, also in the brain) senses this and releases ADH into the bloodstream. When the ADH reaches the kidneys, ADH opens the kidneys' tubules so more water is reabsorbed into your blood instead of being urinated out (Figure 15-1).

After the water pressure goes back up, the hypothalamus detects this and tells the pituitary gland to stop producing ADH. The ADH in the blood drops, and the tubules in the kidneys close so more of the fluid will flow into the urine. This negative feedback loop ensures that our blood holds the perfect amount of water.

If you drink too much water, the body has a means to urinate out the excess but keep a healthy amount in. As long as you have healthy kidneys and urinate when needed, it is almost impossible to overdose on water, it's but easy to be deficient in water. So drink up!

When you drink tea, coffee, soda pop, or alcohol, ADH production goes down. This interferes with the regulation of water in the body, causing you to urinate out too much water. This leads to dehydration, which affects your health (especially over the long term). So for every ounce of alcohol and for every cup of tea or coffee you consume, you should drink at least 8 additional ounces of water.

Minerals and salts

Foot pain from cramps can be a sign of a mineral deficiency like magnesium, calcium, or potassium.

Magnesium: Magnesium relaxes muscles, so a deficiency can lead to spasms.

Calcium: Calcium allows the actin and myosin filaments in muscles to slide along each other during contraction and relaxation. Without calcium, the filaments can't slide, so the muscles lock up.

Electrolytes (salts, minerals, and sugars): You need a proper electrolyte balance for nerves to function properly. People usually eat more foods with sodium than potassium, and this imbalance can lead to muscles cramping. This is why it is often suggested that people eat a banana (which is high in potassium) if they suffer from foot cramps.

You can be deficient in a mineral even if you are ingesting it. You may have an issue of absorption. If this is the case, you may need to apply the mineral topically so it can be directly absorbed into the tissue through the skin. Feet are a great example of this.

Feet are the most distal aspect of your body, so even if you eat mineral-filled foods and take supplements, the mineral may not reach the tissues of your feet. The tension of muscles in your legs may slow the flow of blood in and waste out, contributing to the difficulty getting minerals to the feet. Plus, the weight of your body on your feet makes it difficult to feed the squished tissues of the bottom of your feet.

Topical creams may be a good option for getting minerals to foot tissues. Check out magnesium creams for leg and foot cramps, available on Amazon.

Vitamins

Cramps in the feet can also be a sign of a vitamin deficiency, like Vitamin D, which is necessary for calcium absorption, or Vitamin B2, which is important for nerve health. A deficiency in B2 can lead to nerve pain in the feet.

There has been much debate over whether people should take vitamins. If you are eating a healthy, varied, and whole-foods diet, you should be able to get all of your needed vitamins through your food. Unfortunately, most of our food is grown on over-farmed land, so the food produced on it is deficient of micronutrients and genetically designed to look good and have a longer shelf life (with no to an adverse effect to its nutritional content or taste).

My general advice is to take a half dose of a multivitamin every day or two. That way you are less likely to be deficient in anything and you avoid the risk of overdosing on anything.

If you are taking a multivitamin, make sure the vitamins are coming from a plant source. Plants build vitamins via complex biochemical processes, producing one specific biomolecule. When vitamins are produced in a lab, an unnatural (and potentially harmful) form can be produced and included in the multivitamin pill.

For example, vitamin E has two forms of isomers: an L-alpha tocopherol and a D-alpha tocopherol. Isomers are chemicals that are the same but mirror images of each other. Sometimes this doesn't matter. For example, a cube is the same as its mirror image. But some shapes are such that the mirror image is different from the original. An example of this would be your hands. There is a left (L) and a right (D).

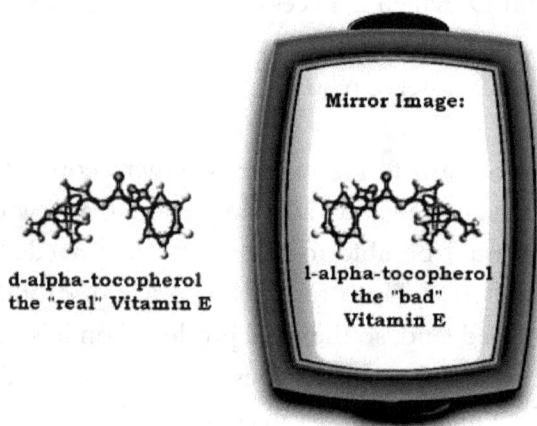

d-alpha-tocopherol
the "real" Vitamin E

Mirror Image:

l-alpha-tocopherol
the "bad"
Vitamin E

Figure 15-2

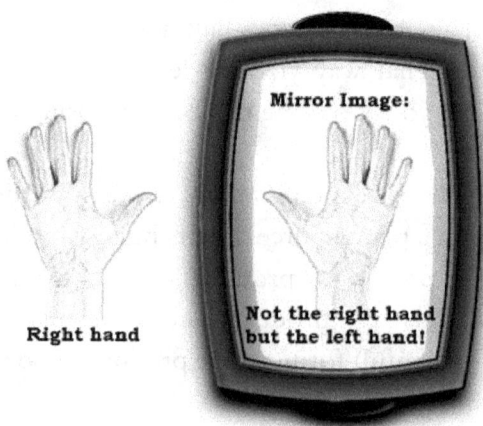

Right hand

Mirror Image:

Not the right hand
but the left hand!

Figure 15-3

Vitamin E has a left and a right version. In Figure 15-2, notice how the carbon cyclohexane (the circle of dots on the far-right side of the molecule) points forward on the D version and points back on the L version.

Do you see how the mirror image is not the same as the original item?

Only the right-hand version of vitamin E, d-alpha tocopherol, works in your body. To help you understand why one works and one doesn't, even though they look similar, think of a lock and key. If the key is just a little bit different, it won't work.

Consider the example of a high-tech lock that is opened by your unique right hand. Let's say you can only open it by inserting your right-hand so it can read your fingerprints. Your left hand wouldn't be able to open it. Even if your left hand had the exact same fingerprints as your right hand, it still wouldn't be able to open the lock because the fingerprints would be in the wrong order and the thumb would be on the wrong side.

That's what happens with the left and right vitamin E. The right one works, but the left one doesn't. An easy way to remember this is "L is for liar."

Look at your vitamin label. If it says the vitamin E is dl-alpha tocopherol, it has the unnatural form of vitamin E as well as the natural version (hence the d and the l). In my opinion, you should throw this away because it may be harmful to your health. Look for a multivitamin that has the d-alpha tocopherol version instead.

If you take a calcium supplement, make sure it also has vitamin D (for better absorption) and magnesium (which is good for muscle cramps and helps prevent constipation, which can occur with taking calcium).

Talk to your healthcare providers to see what is best for your individual needs.

Chapter 16: MEDICATION, DRUGS, CHEMICALS AND FOOT PAIN

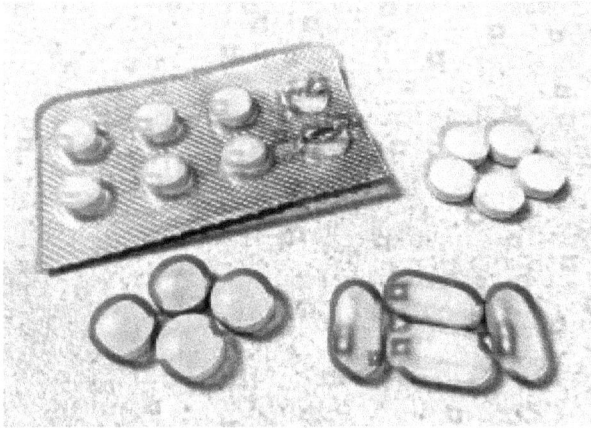

S OME PRESCRIPTION MEDICATIONS can result in foot pain as a side effect.

Cholesterol-lowering medications, called statins, can cause muscle and joint pain, including those of the lower extremity.

Chemotherapy drugs can cause peripheral nerve damage, meaning the distal ends of the nerves (like those in your feet) are harmed by these drugs, and can cause pain.

Opioids (Pain-Relieving Drugs)

Yes, taking powerful pain-relieving drugs can actually result in more pain! Taking opioids over time decreases your body's ability to handle pain, making the pain feel even worse when the medication wears off. Plus, the body learns to break down the medication, making it less effective over time. This can make you more dependent on these drugs. Even taking over-the-counter (OTC) pain relievers can result in rebound pain and dependency.

Why an Easy Solution Can Be Harmful

When people have foot pain, the first thing they usually reach for is an everyday painkiller like ibuprofen or aspirin. However, nonsteroidal anti-inflammatory drugs (NSAIDs), like acetaminophen, ibuprofen, or aspirin, are not as safe to take as many people think. Such drugs have side effects and are very hard on the liver and kidneys, and can lead to organ failure and early death.

Indeed, I know people who take several OTC pain relievers every day and have for years. But some people get away with smoking for years, too, and never develop cancer or COPD (chronic obstructive pulmonary disease). This does not mean smoking is safe. In the same way, people who take pain relievers every day do so at a cost to their overall health.

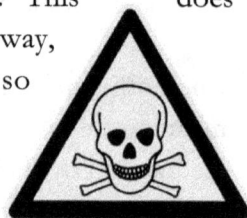

Don't get me wrong. I'm grateful to have access to medicines; they definitely have their uses. But America has a problem with overprescribing drugs. As an example, 99 percent of the world's Vicodin is prescribed in the United States.[1]

I have treated many people who were taking so many medications that they had to keep a written list of them. Some of these drugs were prescribed to treat the side effects of the medications they were taking for their original complaint. Sadly, instead of curing their condition, the medications were muting the symptoms of their disease. After educating these patients about lifestyle changes and herbal remedies, I helped them get off many of their medications (with their medical doctor's approval).

Medication is great for the short term because it offers a quick fix, but long-term use of chemicals is unhealthy. Prolonged use of medication leads to a decrease in quality of life. Such patients may be living with less pain, but at what cost to their body?

Consider this startling statistic: "NSAID use causes nearly 103,000 hospitalizations and 16,500 deaths. More people die each year from NSAIDs-related complications than from AIDS and cervical cancer in the US."[2] Furthermore, I have had too many patients in their late sixties find out that they have

---

[1] Vicodin Addiction. "Nearly 100 Percent of the World's Vicodin Prescriptions Are Used in U.S." Vicodin Addiction."
[2] American Gastroenterological Association, "Study Shows Long-term Use of NSAIDs Causes Severe Intestinal Damage."

stage three kidney failure because of their NSAID usage over the years. And I have known of too many people who have died of liver failure because of acetaminophen usage.[3]

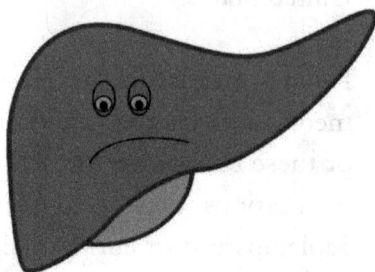

Why Avoiding Pain Relievers Is a Better Solution

So how do you balance the speed of pain relief that NSAIDs bring with their potential harmful effects? First, try other treatments to relieve your discomfort. If you take pain pills every day, their effectiveness wears off over time, and eventually you will have a difficult time overcoming the pain, even with pain relievers.

I do not believe in masking pain—we have pain for a reason. You do not want to turn off your body's alarm system. It would be like taking the battery out of the fire alarms in your home so you don't have to listen to them beep as your house burns down.

If you are not suffering from a traumatic injury but from chronic aches and pains, finding the root source of the pain and treating it through diet, stretches, and exercises instead of masking the pain is far healthier in the long run.

---

[3] Zimmerman, "Drugs Used to Treat Rheumatic and Musculospastic Disease," *Hepatotoxicity*.

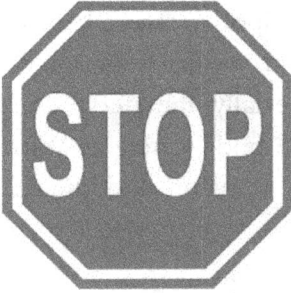

If you are taking pain relievers regularly, *stop*!

The fast and easy path for relieving foot pain is to take pain medication, but it is also the path to a shorter lifespan.

Yes, you will feel *awful* for a few weeks as you find other ways to treat your foot pain, but tough it out. Once your body re-acclimates to a healthier lifestyle, you will rarely be in pain, and even if you are in pain, you may not need pain relievers to alleviate it.

If you take pain pills for every ache and pain, I hope this book persuades you to try other treatments. I often hear from new patients that they take over-the-counter pain relievers almost every day for their foot pain! After they learn to support their feet, stretch and move their feet more often throughout the day, eat healthier, avoid high impact activities, and self-massage their feet, they often find they no longer need to take pain relievers.

So instead of pain relievers, check out the following treatments for your foot pain, and talk to your healthcare provider to see what would be best for your individual needs.

Cigarette Smoking

The drugs and chemicals found in cigarettes damage the lining of the blood vessels, causing them to thicken and narrow, raising your blood pressure. The delicate vessels of the capillary beds are grossly affected by the higher blood pressure because it affects the transfer of nutrients and wastes between the tissues and blood. Foot tissues (especially the nerves) are already under the stress of bearing the body's weight. Marry this stressor with the damage caused by smoking, and it makes sense that foot pain results.

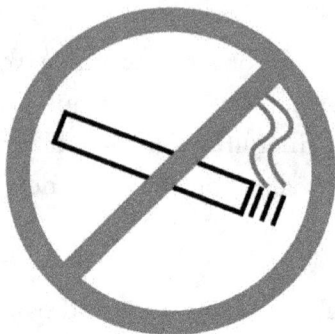

Yet another reason to not smoke.

Chapter 17: SHOES – WHAT YOU DON'T KNOW CAN HURT YOU

BASICALLY PUT, healthy feet are a result of good support, lack of injury, good nutrition, good genetics, and good hygiene. In this chapter, we are going to focus on what to avoid and what to look for in shoes.

Poor Shoes

Some people believe less support is better. They talk about how it's not natural to wear shoes, and that doing so makes the muscles in our feet weaker.

These are my thoughts on such claims.

I agree, it is not natural to wear shoes. But I also realize it is not natural to walk on hard, flat surfaces all day. If we were running around outside on natural, soft, uneven surfaces, then yes, we should all be barefoot.

However, most of us walk on at worst concrete floors or, at best, carpeted floors. If we don't wear shoes with arch supports, our poor feet are subjected to unnatural forces that sprain or strain our arches over time, leading to collapsed arches, plantar fasciitis, and/or heel spurs.

Plus, the extra cushion found in good shoes helps pad the blow of our heel striking the ground, which saves our knees, hips, and back from the jarring forces that otherwise lead to their early degeneration.

To know what shoes are good for your specific needs, you first have to understand your feet. As mentioned in Chapter 3, your feet may be over-pronating, supinating, or positioned neutrally (Figure 17-1).

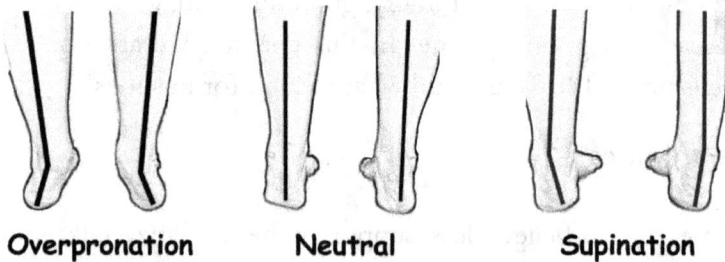

Overpronation   **Neutral**   **Supination**

Figure 17-1

If your feet overpronate, you need orthotics that will support your arches and help control the motion of your gait.

If your feet supinate, you will need more cushion because your higher rigid arches don't absorb as much shock as they should. You may also need high arch supports to prevent your arches from collapsing.

If your feet are healthy, keep them that way by supporting them with good-fitting supportive shoes.

Arch Type	Foot Alignment	Shoe Type
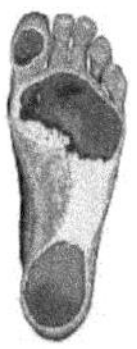 Normal Arch	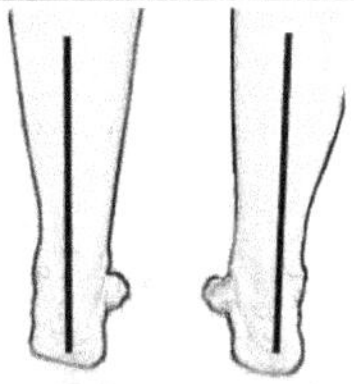 Neutral	STABILITY SHOE
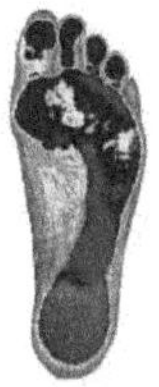 High Arch	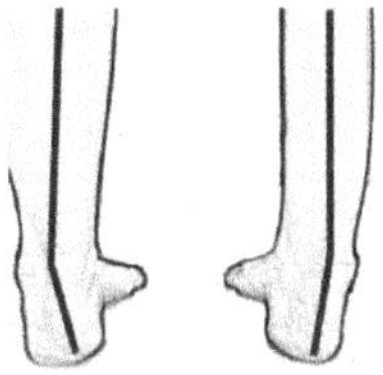 Supination	CUSHIONED SHOE
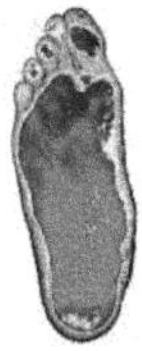 Flat Feet	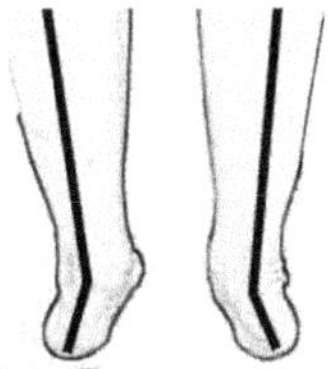 Over-Pronation	MOTION CONTROL SHOE

Figure 17-2: Different feet need different shoes and insoles.

Understanding your feet will help you determine the type of shoe that is perfect for your needs (Figure 17-2).

With this said, watch out for shoes that have a bubble of extra support in the heel (Figure 17-3).

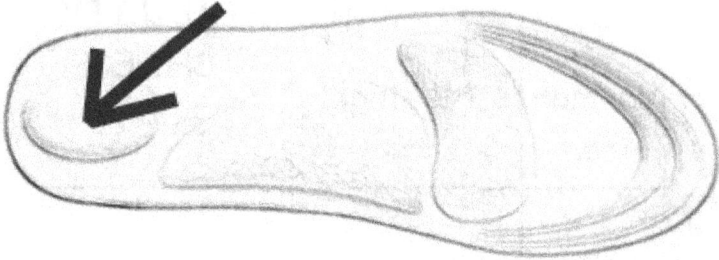

Figure 17-3: Example of an insert with a bump in the heel region.

Having extra cushion under the heel may sound like a good idea, but this often causes more pressure to be exerted on the heel bone, leading to heel pain. The pressure of the bubble can irritate the tendon of the plantar muscles or the plantar ligaments (like the plantar fascia), causing them to be rubbed raw. This can result in plantar fasciitis or heel spurs.

I prefer a hallowed-out area for the heel (Figure 17-4). That way the pressure is shifted to the edges of the heel bone, instead of placed on the center where the plantar fascia anchors.

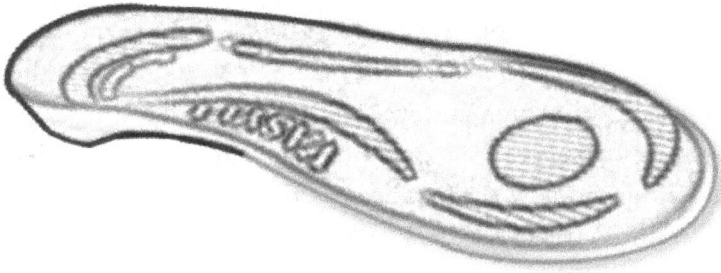

Figure 17-4: An insert with a hollowed-out heel.

High heels

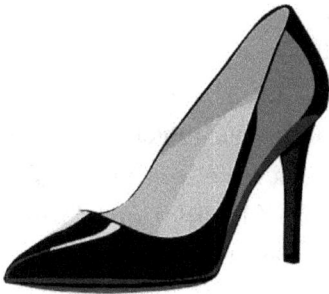

I hope it is obvious how wearing high heels puts stress on your feet, ankles, knees, and muscles of the feet and lower legs. But it also causes your pelvis to tilt forward and compresses your low back, which can cause hip and low back pain.

I have had patients who came in to be treated for low back pain that was caused by wearing high heels at work for so many years. They thought they could only wear high heels because their lower legs hurt when they wore flat shoes. Wearing heels for so long caused their calf muscles to shorten, so they could no longer bring their heels to the ground. Wearing flats became impossibly uncomfortable, so they wore heels all the time, making their over-shortened calf muscles even shorter. Eventually they developed low back pain.

If you never bring your heel to the ground, one day you won't be able to. Remember, if you don't use it, you lose it.

With daily stretching and wearing incrementally shorter heels, these patients were able to stretch their calf muscles enough to where they could wear flats again. Once they were able to wear flatter shoes, their low back pain went away.

Flip-flops

Any shoe that makes you change your normal gait puts abnormal stressors on your body. Flip-flops fall into this category.

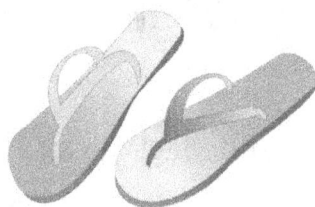

You have a big calf muscle in the back of your lower leg to toe off. When you wear flip-flops, your toes have to grip to hold the shoe on, and you excessively toe up (dorsiflexion) during the gait cycle, causing the flip-flop action. This action strains the front lower muscles (the muscles that raise your toes and forefoot), which can lead to foot, ankle, knee, hip, and back pain.

To be fair, a study was done in Australia that showed wearing flip-flops was closer to being barefoot than we originally thought. But in my book, it's close, but no cigar. I have had too many patients with foot and lower leg complaints who felt better when they stopped wearing flip-flops.

My One Exception to Wearing Flip-Flops...

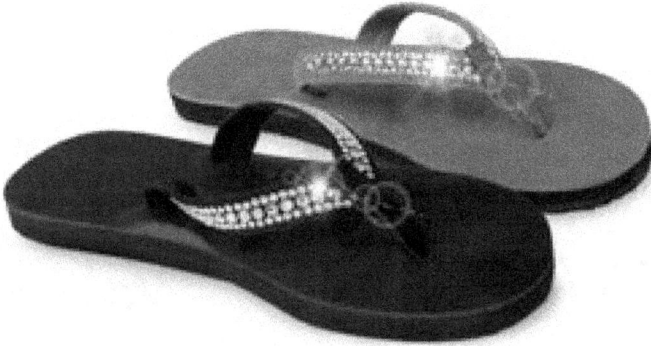

Figure 17-5: Foot Leveler Flip-Flops.

Every rule has an exception, and my rules are not exempt. Foot Levelers has a flip-flop orthotic that I prescribe for patients who need an easy-to-slip-on shoe to wear while doing dishes or other household activities that do not involve a lot of walking (Figures 17-5 and 17-6). Better to stand on a Foot Leveler flip-flop orthotic than stand unsupported on a hard floor.

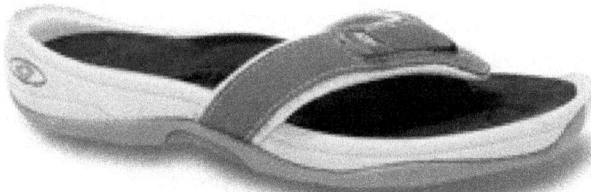

Figure 17-6: Foot Leveler Supportive Flip-Flop.

If you are going to go for a walk in your sandals, a better option is to wear a sandal orthotic with a heel strap (Figure 17-6). This will prevent the flip-flop action, allowing for a more natural gait.

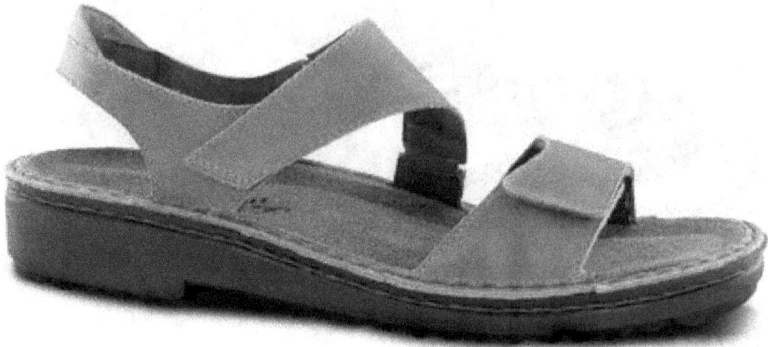

Figure 17-7: Sandal orthotic you can walk in (has a heel strap).

What Makes a Good-Fitting Shoe?

I've talked about the shoes you shouldn't wear if you want to have healthy feet. Here's what you should look for in a pair of shoes.

Plenty of room for the toes

Many people wear shoes that are too small. Your feet continue to grow as you age, so double-check your shoe size periodically. You can tell if your shoes are big enough by simply taking out the shoes' insoles and standing on them. Your feet should fit inside the edges of the insoles. If any part of your foot hangs over an edge—whether it's the tip of a toe or the side of your foot—the shoes are too small. Many times this test has revealed that the shoes my patients were wearing were too small by a half size or more.

Plus, some people have a longer second toe. Most shoes are designed for a longer first toe. If your second toe is longer, the shoe's shape may cause it to bend, causing hammer, mallet, or claw toe of the second toe (as discussed in Chapter 7).

Plenty of room for the forefoot

Most shoes are designed with a narrowing of the forefoot (Figure 17-8). This design can be uncomfortable for people whose forefoot is wider than their heel.

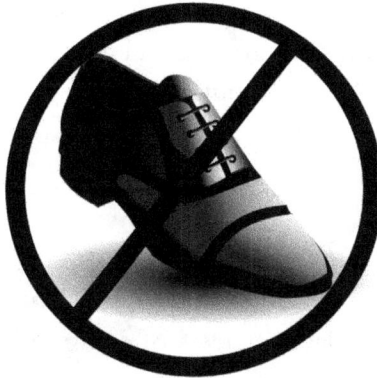

Figure 17-8: Avoid shoes with a narrow toe box (hard on toes).

Again, standing on the insole should help determine if the shoe's toe box is wide enough for your toes.

If you like the look of a shoe that narrows in the forefoot, you may be able to wear the shoe but in a larger size.

Orthotics and shoe size

One thing I love about being professionally fit for orthotics is it makes shoe sizing easy. You have to take the insoles out of your shoes to make room for the orthotics. When you put the orthotics in the shoe, if the orthotics don't fit in the shoes, then the shoes are not the right fit for your feet.

Plus, you can buy cheaper shoes, as the expense of the shoe is often due to the insole. You can get a cheaper shoe with a cheap insole, as you are going to replace it with your custom professionally made insoles.

High impact activities on hard surfaces—a double negative

If your job requires you to stand all day, especially on concrete floors, invest in extra padding in your shoes, and see about getting thick rubber mats to lay down in spots where you stand most frequently.

If you have read any of my other books, you know I don't like to blame age for health problems, but I have to admit, some things are unavoidable aspects of aging. As we get older, our subcutaneous fat thins. This is why our skin wrinkles as we age. In our feet, the fat pad under our heels is made of subcutaneous fat, so it thins as we age. This makes our heel bones more sensitive to hard surfaces as we get older. It just doesn't seem fair that we lose fat where we need it and gain it where we don't want it!

Chapter 18: PROPRIOCEPTION AND FOOT PAIN

T HIS CHAPTER EXPLAINS what proprioception is, how poor proprioception can cause foot pain, and how to improve proprioception to help alleviate foot pain.

Proprioception

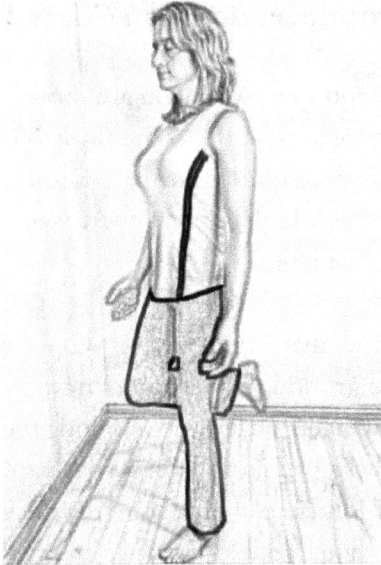

Figure 18-1

We are visual creatures and rely on our vision to tell us where we are in our surroundings. To help us determine what our body is doing in space, mechanisms in our inner ears tell our brains how we are moving. Yet, even with our eyes closed and when we are still, we know where our hands and feet are. This is because we have nerve fibers throughout our body that give our brains even more input as to where we are in space. Our awareness of where we are in space is called proprioception.

Most people lose their balance as they age. I attribute this to the fact that many people do not exercise their balance. How often do you stand on one foot with your eyes closed? Again, if you don't use it, you lose it.

How Poor Proprioception Can Cause Foot Pain

If your proprioception is poor, you are more likely to misjudge where your feet are in relation to the floor. This results in your feet hitting the ground harder during your heel strike while you walk. This repetitive high impact increases your risk of hip, knee, heel, and foot pain.

Have you noticed that when some people walk, their heels loudly strike the ground, while others have very quiet strikes? The louder your heels strike the ground, the harder you are hitting it, and the more jarring forces you are subjecting your heel bones and joints to with each step. Try to walk softer. Your body will thank you for it. Walking more softly is easier to do if you have a strong sense of proprioception.

How to Measure and Improve Your Proprioception

To measure your body's proprioception, you need to remove the other two indicators of your body's position: sight and detection of movement by your inner ears. You can do this by closing your eyes (to remove the visual reference) and standing still on one leg (without movement, your inner ears aren't much assistance). You should do this by a wall or with your hands hovering over a counter so you can prevent yourself from falling if you start to wobble too much (Figure 18-2).

You should be able to do this for at least thirty seconds per leg (three minutes if you are an athlete). If you can't, then you are vulnerable to injury if you get visually distracted and misstep. Good proprioception allows you to catch yourself from falling, making you less likely to twist an ankle (or, when you're elderly, break a bone). If you don't practice your proprioception, you are more likely to fall without grace, resulting in injury.

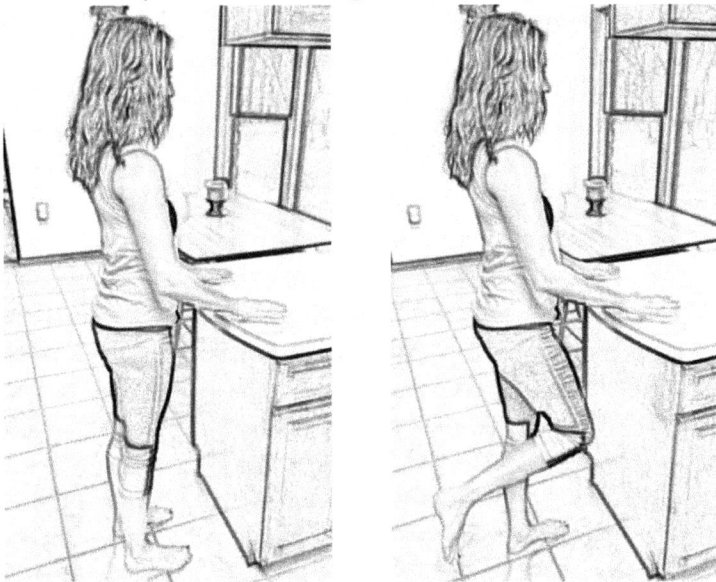

Figure 18-2: Working on proprioception while hovering my hands over a counter, eyes closed, and standing with one foot off the floor.

To improve your proprioception, stand on one leg with your eyes closed and your hands near something you can grab once or twice a day. Once you can comfortably stand on one leg with your eyes closed for thirty seconds, you may be able to do this exercise next to a wall, making it easier to do throughout the day.

Everyone should do this exercise every day. People sit too much, often with poor posture. If you don't fight the effects of sitting, you become more bent and stiff with time. Your brain doesn't notice this slow decline, but when you reach that tipping point, you start misjudging where you are in space to such a degree that you become clumsy. I have had patients who started having multiple falls in situations where they shouldn't, for example, when going from carpet to hard flooring. Once they worked on their proprioception, they didn't fall as often (if at all).

With improved proprioception, you should naturally walk lighter on your feet, taking the stressors away that may be causing your foot pain.

In the meantime, walk with more cushion in your shoes, and take time throughout the day to consciously walk light on your feet.

Chapter 19: EXERCISES AND STRETCHES FOR FOOT PAIN

T HIS CHAPTER EXPLAINS how to strengthen the muscles of the lower extremities to help support the foot and stretch the muscles and joints of the lower legs and feet to help alleviate foot pain.

To stabilize a region, strengthen the muscles in front, behind, and on both sides of the joint needing stability. Strengthening all four quadrants will improve stability because the muscles will hold the joint in place when it experiences unstabilizing forces from any direction.

This chapter includes exercises for the muscles in front, behind, inside, outside, above, and below the knee. Strengthening these muscles will stabilize the ankle and foot, making them less vulnerable to injury.

Heel Lifts and Toe Lifts

Heel and toe lifts strengthen the lower leg muscles. Heel lifts strengthen the calf muscles in the back, and toe lifts strengthen the muscles in the front of the lower leg.

While standing, rise up on your toes and lower back down. Then lift your toes up, balancing on your heels, and lower them back down. Keep repeating this rocking motion several times (Figure 19-1). This will also act as a pump to aid lymph flow out of the lower extremities.

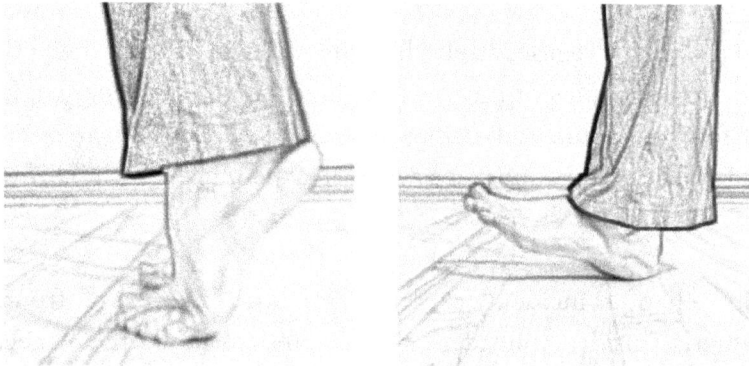

Figure 19-1: Heel and Toe Lifts

Strengthening the Muscles in Your Feet with Toe Curls

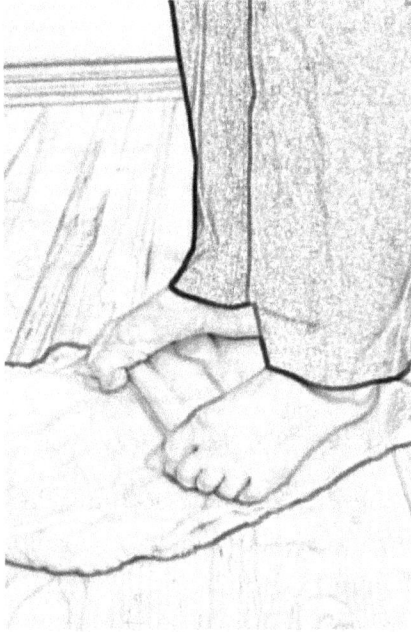

Figure 19-2: Toe Curls

Toe curls can be done seated or standing, and even while you are wearing shoes.

If you have on shoes, curl your toes to squeeze the material of your socks between your toes.

If you're barefoot, use a towel as shown in Figure 19-2. This exercises the plantar muscles of the feet. Repeat several times. This strengthens the foot muscles and helps pump the excess fluids out of your lower extremities as well.

Strengthening lower leg muscles with an exercise band

Eversion for lateral (outer) lower leg strengthening

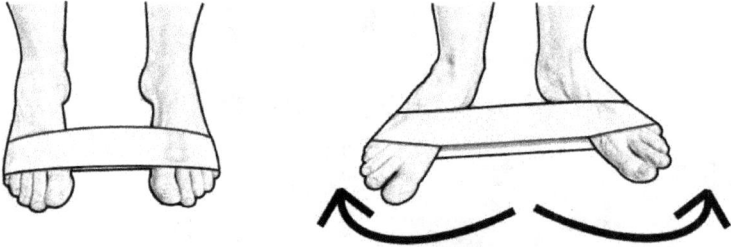

Figure 19-3: Neutral to Eversion

To strengthen the lateral lower leg muscles (the peroneus muscles), sit down in a chair and put the rubber band around your forefeet (Figure 19-3). Keeping your heels in place, press your feet outward (an action called eversion).

This strengthens the peroneus muscles, which support the lateral arch of the foot.

Inversion for medial (inner) lower leg strengthening

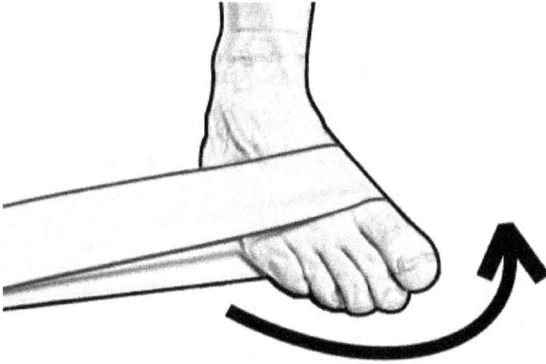

Figure 19-4: Inversion Exercise

To strengthen the medial lower leg muscles (the tibialis muscles), put the rubber band around your forefoot (Figure 19-4), and tether the other end of the rubber band to a heavy chair or table. Keeping your heel in place, press your foot inward (an action called inversion). Perform this exercise in a seated or prone (on your back) position for ease of stability.

This strengthens the tibialis muscles, which support the longitudinal arch of the foot.

STRENGTHENING THE LOWER EXTREMITIES ABOVE THE KNEES HELPS FOOT PAIN TOO

If you have foot pain, further support of the muscles of the thigh is usually needed. If thigh muscles are weak, the lower leg muscles have to compensate, which can be a strain on the feet. The exercises in this section are offered with this in mind.

Quad (Top of Thigh) Strengthening

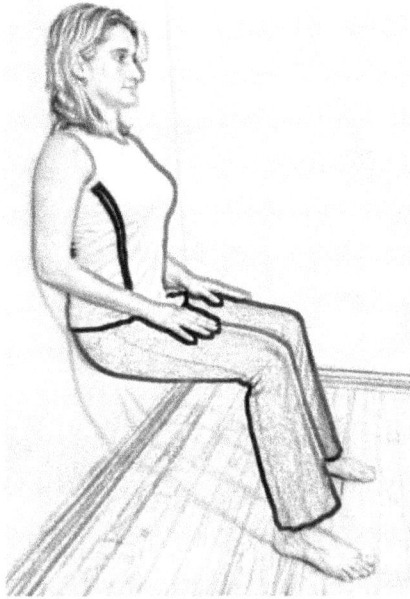

Figure 19-5

To exercise your quadriceps muscles, the muscles in the front of your upper thigh, stand with your back against a wall, walk your feet out farther than the length of your thighs, and squat by sliding your back down the wall (Figure 19-5). Protect your knees by not squatting too deeply; do not allow your knees to go past your feet. Hold this position for five breaths.

This is a great way to strengthen the quads because your back is supported by the wall. It is also a good exercise to repeat throughout the day for leg strengthening, making for a quick calorie burn.

Stronger Quad (Thigh) Strengthening

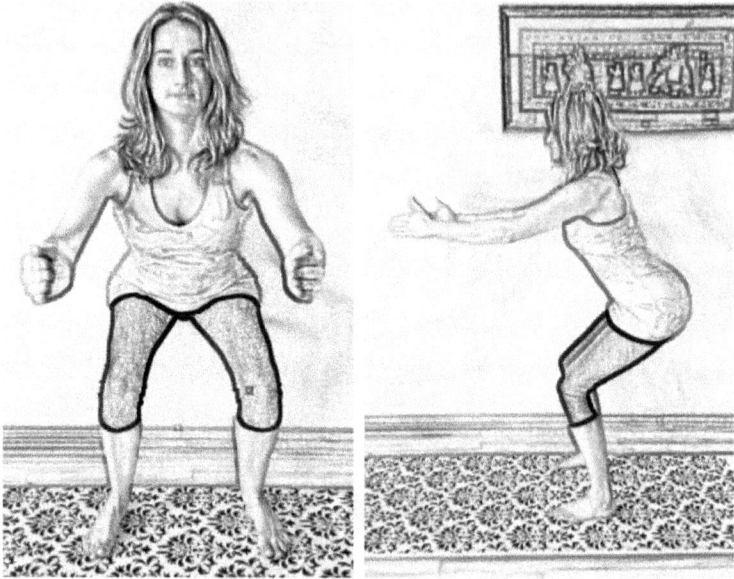

Figure 19-6: Freestanding squats.

After you are able to do wall squats comfortably, try doing freestanding squats.

Stand with your feet shoulder width apart. Then extend your arms in front of you and move your buttocks back as if you're going to sit in a chair (Figure 19-6). Make sure your knees don't move forward in front of your feet because this can strain the knees.

Work toward repeating a dozen times, and then repeat this several times throughout the day. You can do this exercise anywhere, and it doesn't take long to do. Again, the frequency—not the intensity or duration—is what's important to build strength and combat the effects of sitting too much.

After you've mastered freestanding squats, try going even lower with your squats (Figure 19-7).

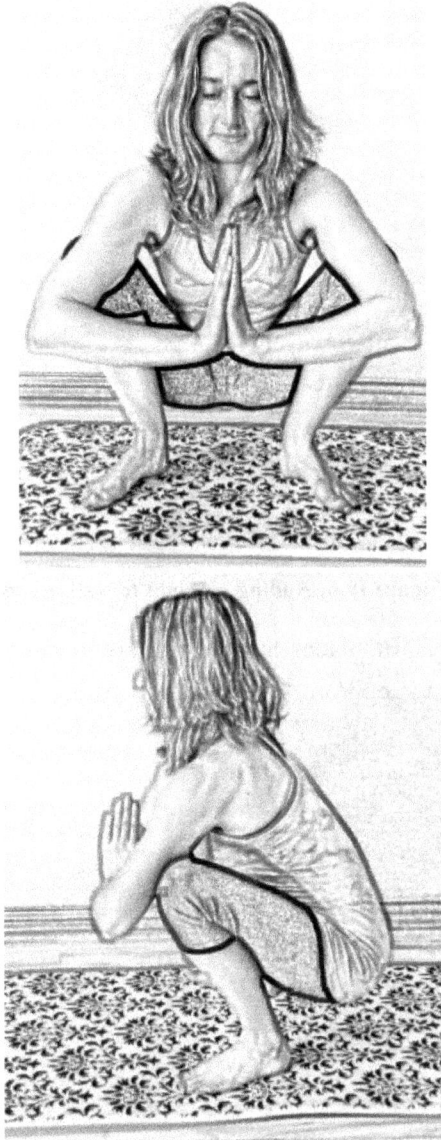

Figure 19-7: Deep squats.

For an even more intense quad workout, add a weight to your thighs while doing a wall squat (Figure 19-8).

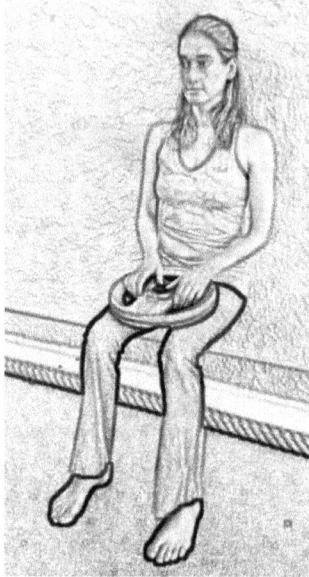

Figure 19-8: Adding a weight to wall squats.

The added weight places even more strain on your knees, so make sure you keep your knees behind your toes and over your heels.

Adductor (Inside Thigh) Strengthening

To work the inside thigh muscles, place a ball between your knees while you are doing a wall squat (Figure 19-9). Squeezing your knees against the ball will strengthen the adductor muscles.

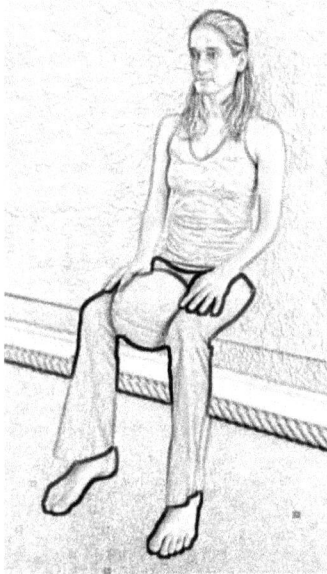

Figure 19-9: Squeeze a ball between your knees to strengthen your thigh muscles.

An alternative is to lie on your left side, bend your right knee, and place your right foot behind your left leg (Figure 19-10).

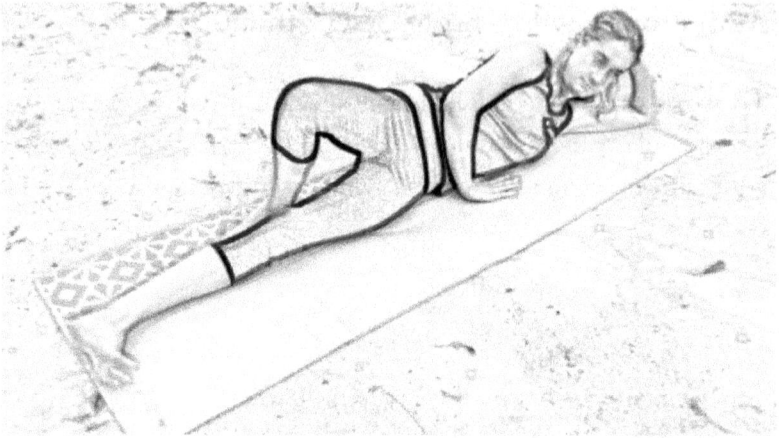

Figure 19-10: The starting position for adductor muscle strengthening.

Support your head with your left hand. Stabilize yourself by placing your right hand on the ground. Keep your pelvis perpendicular to the ground and protect your low back by keeping your spine in line. Don't allow your right hip to roll back or forward. Keep your right foot on the ground behind you. Flex your left foot so your toes lift toward your head.

Now you are in a position to work out your left adductor muscle. To do so, contract your inner left thigh by lifting your left foot away from the ground (Figure 19-11). If you feel your front or back thigh muscles engaging, you are not in the correct position.

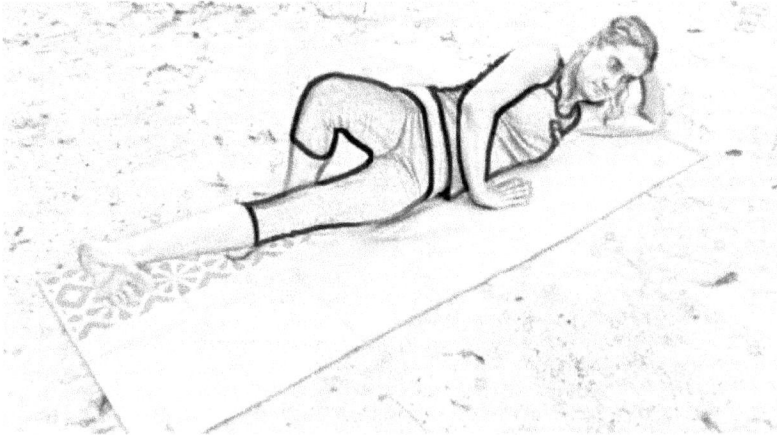

Figure 19-11: Contracting the left adductor muscle.

Exercise your left thigh by repeating this exercise a few times, and then roll over and exercise your right thigh.

Strengthening the adductor muscles helps stabilize the ankles, knees, hips and pelvis, making your feet and ankles less vulnerable to injury.

TFL (Outside Thigh) Strengthening

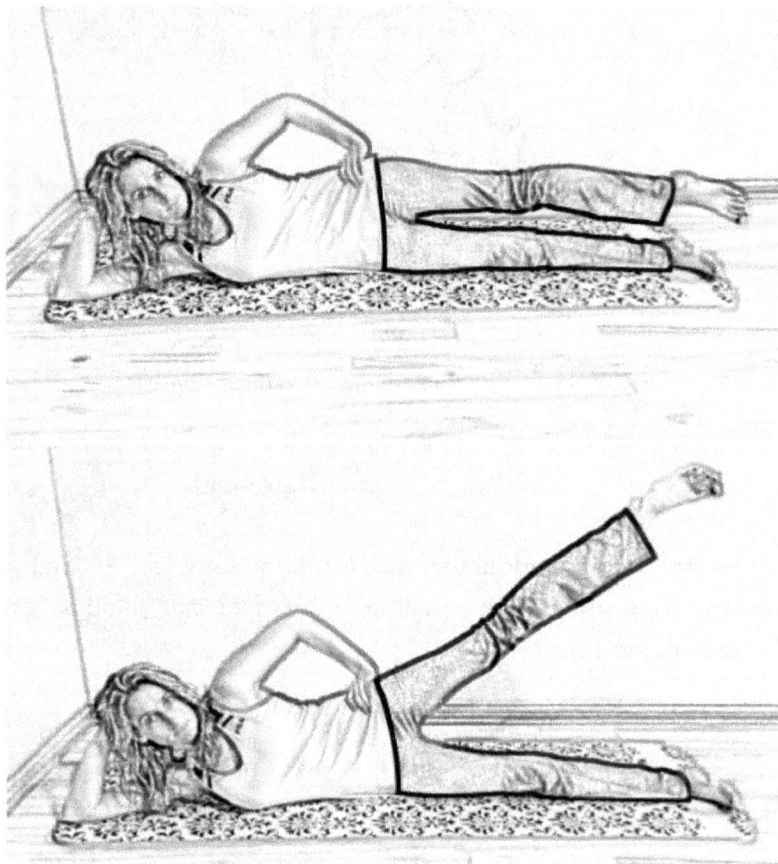

Figure 19-12: Side leg raises to strengthen the TFL.

To exercise the muscles on the outside of your thighs, lie on your right side. Keep your hips perpendicular to the floor (one hip on top of the other). Raise your left hip. Keep your toes pointed toward your face as you lift your left leg. Pause at your farthest point for a breath or two (Figure 19-12). Then lower your left leg and pause for a breath or two just before it touches the right leg. Repeat three to ten times. Then repeat on the other side.

To increase resistance and make this exercise more difficult, put a mini loop exercise band just above your ankles (Figure 19-13). You can buy a set of mini loop exercise bands online for under $10.

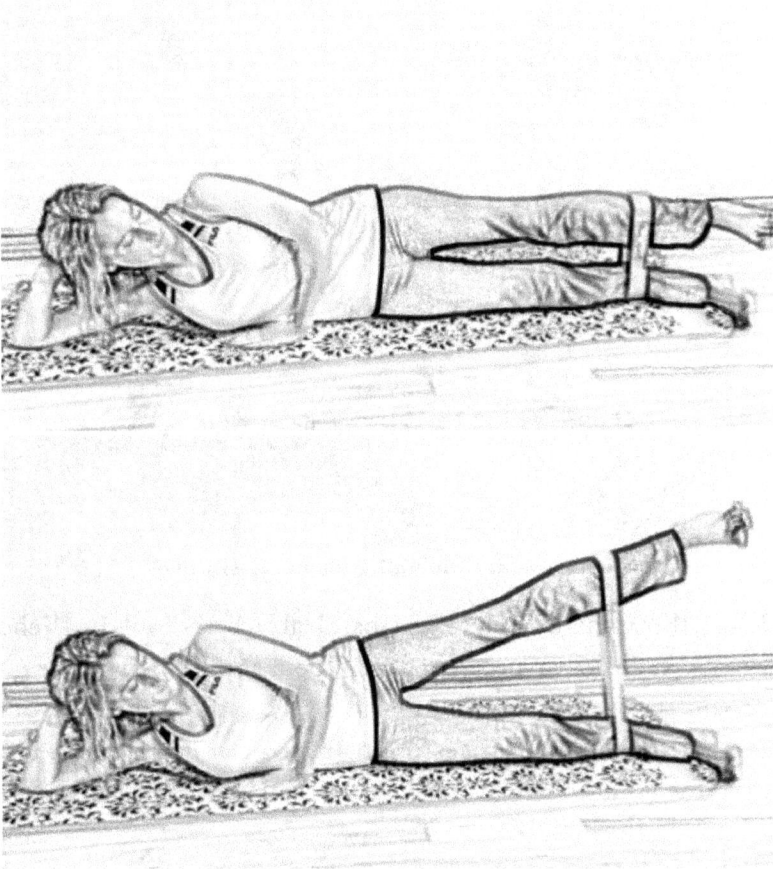

Figure 19-13: Side leg raise with an exercise band.

Perform the same movements as described in the previous TFL exercise. The band will make it more intense.

You can also work out your TFL muscles using the mini loop exercise band while standing.

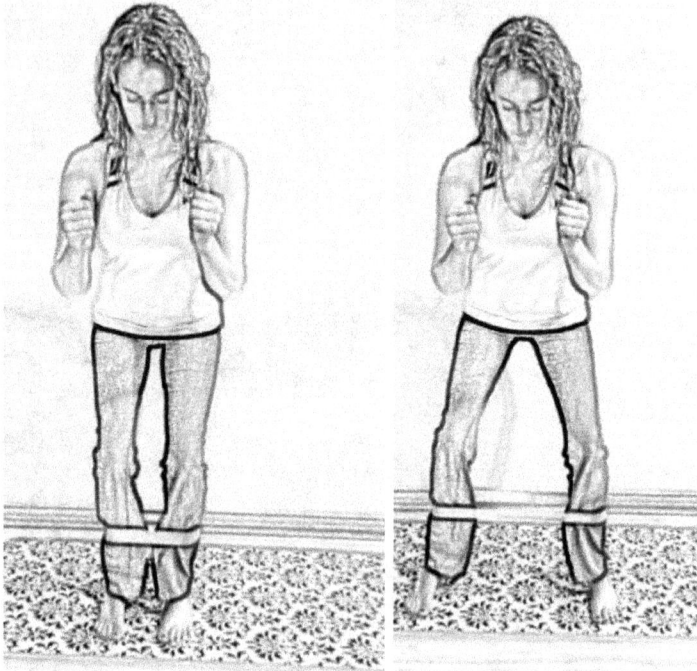

Figure 19-14: Crab walk with an exercise band.

Place the mini loop exercise band above the ankles. Bend slightly at the waist; hold your arms, bent at the elbows, in front of your body; and keep your knees above the arches of your feet. If you let your knees go in front of your feet, you risk harming your knees.

Move your left leg sideways away from your right leg as far as you can and then plant your left foot on the mat (Figure 19-14). Move your right foot back to your left foot and repeat. You will slowly move to your left. Sometimes this exercise is referred to as the crab walk.

When you have moved as far as you want to go, reverse, and walk sideways back to your start position. Repeat three times.

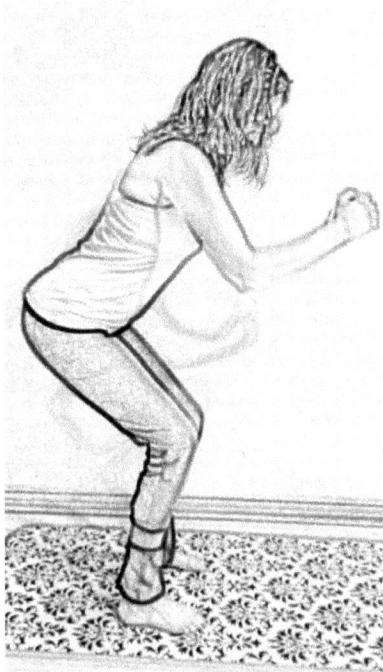

Figure 19-15: Crab walk from the side view.

Again, note how the knees are over the arches of the feet while doing the crab walk (Figure 9-11). Keep your knees behind your toes because you don't want to hurt your knees while trying to help your feet.

Combining TFL Strengthening with Core Strengthening

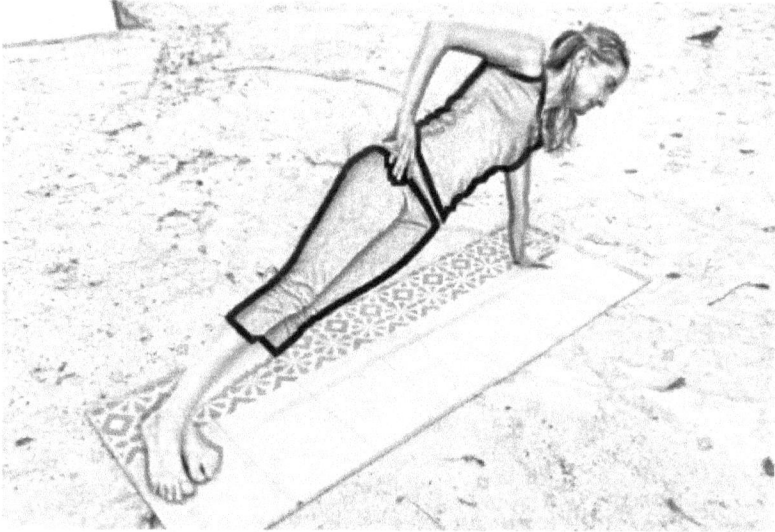

Figure 19-16: A basic side plank.

A side plank (Figure 19-16) is a great way to strengthen the lateral thigh muscles and your core muscles at the same time.

Get into a side plank by starting in a plank position. Place your left hand under your nose, then turn to the right so the lateral aspect your left foot is on the ground and your right foot rests on top of your left foot. Make sure your left hand is placed under your shoulder, your left wrist is in a comfortable position, and your body alignment is straight (so your pelvic bones are on top of each other, not tilted forward or backward).

If this is too difficult, you can rest your left knee on the ground as in Figure 19-17.

An Easier Side Plank

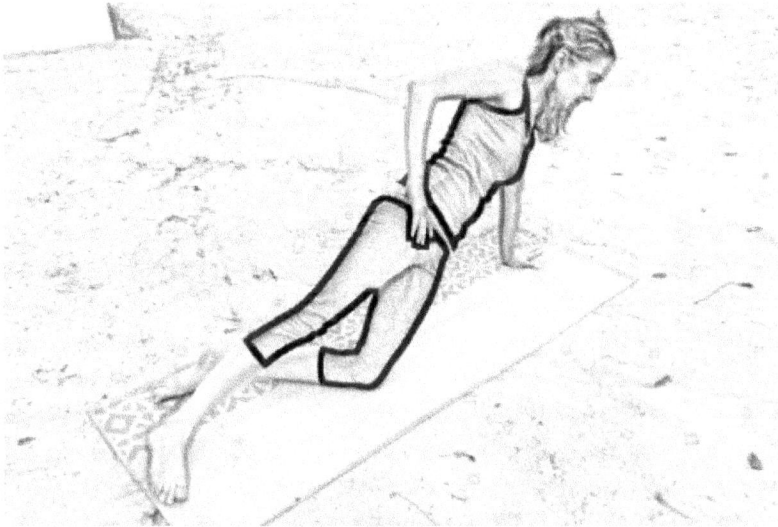

Figure 19-17: Modified Side Plank.

If placing the weight of your upper body on your arm causes wrist pain, you can hold this position from your left forearm instead of your left wrist. Simply rest the side of your forearm from your elbow to your wrist and the side of your hand on the ground.

A Harder Side Plank

To make this more intense for your TFL, raise your top leg. To really work your core at the same time, raise your top arm (Figure 9-18).

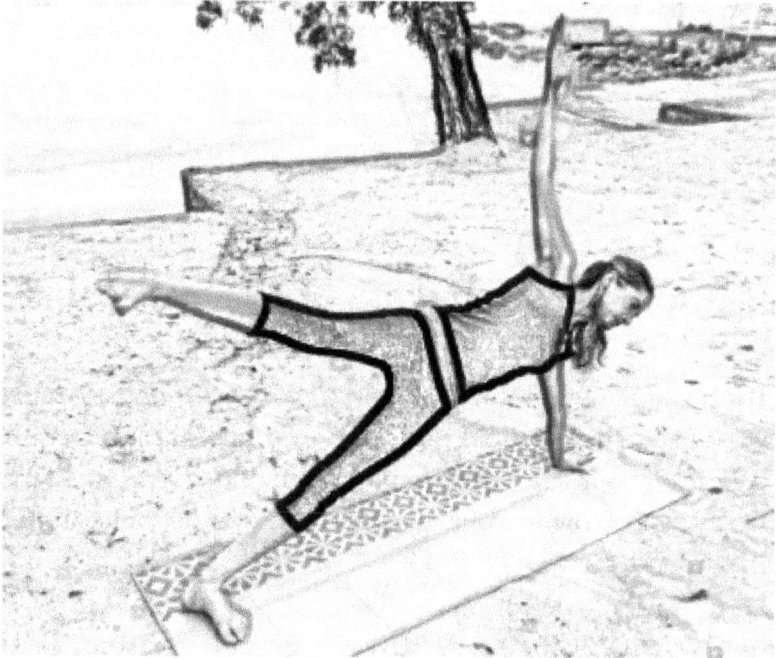

Figure 19-18: An advanced side plank.

Hamstring (Back of Thigh) Strengthening

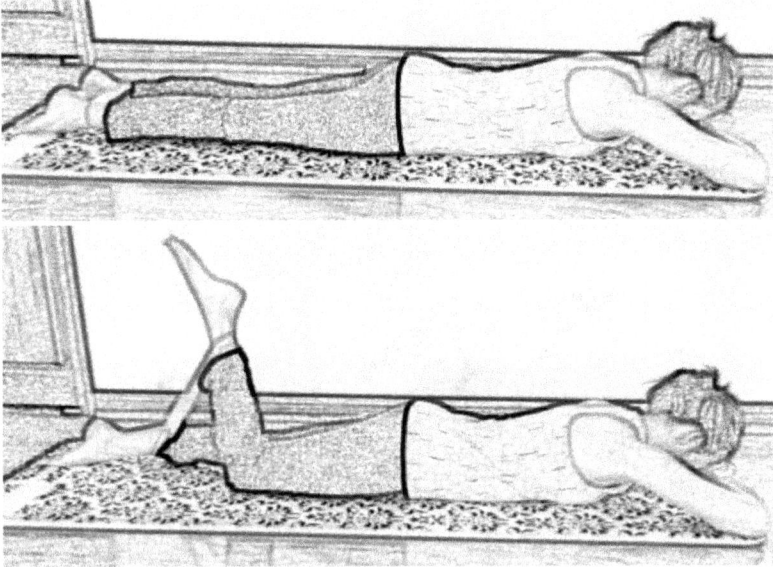

Figure 19-19: Strengthening the hamstrings with mini loop bands.

To strengthen the muscles in the back of your thighs, put a mini loop exercise band around your ankles and lie on your stomach. Keep your left leg straight and on the ground as you bend your right knee (Figure 19-19). The resistance from the band will strengthen the right hamstring.

Do three to five right knee bends, and then repeat on the other side. Repeat three times as long as you feel *no* pain in the knee joint. You don't want to sprain your knee while trying to strengthen your hamstrings.

Deep Calf (Back of Lower Leg) and Bottom of Foot Stretch

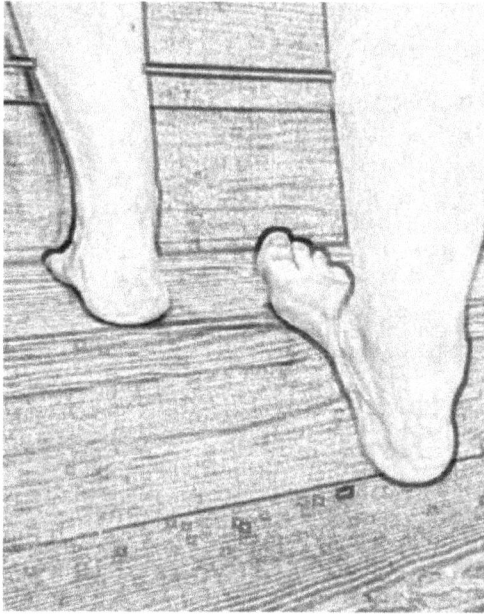

Figure 19-20: Deep Calf Stretch

Facing a stairway going up, stand on the bottom step and hold on to the rail for balance. Bring your right foot back so your toes are at the edge of the step. Keep your weight on your left foot. Allow your right heel to gently extend toward the floor to stretch your right calf (Figure 19-20). Hold for three breaths. Then repeat on the other side.

This exercise can be done with shoes on, unless you are wearing high heels. If you are wearing high heels, use this stretch as an opportunity to take them off for a minute. Be sure to wiggle your toes before doing this stretch.

Calf Stretches Continued

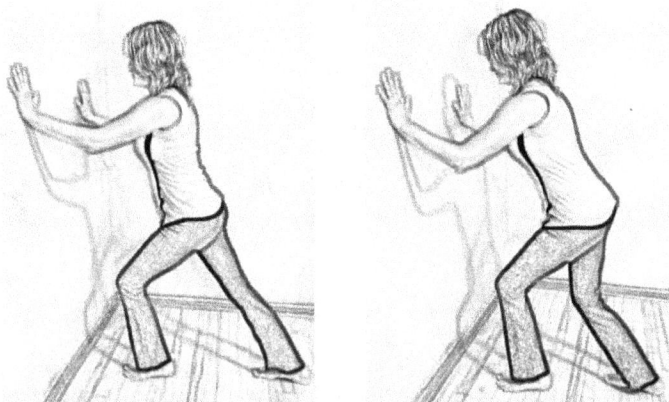

Figure 19-21

To stretch the calf muscles in the back of your lower leg, stand facing a wall and put your hands against the wall. Bring your right leg back and stretch your right heel toward the floor (this stretches the gastrocnemius muscle at the back of your calf, connected to the Achilles tendon). Hold for three breaths. Then bend your right knee to stretch the soleus muscle (the deeper muscle under the gastrocnemius). Hold for three breaths.

Repeat on the other side.

This not only stretches the muscles of the calf, but of the arches of the feet.

Foot ABCs for Lymphatic Drainage

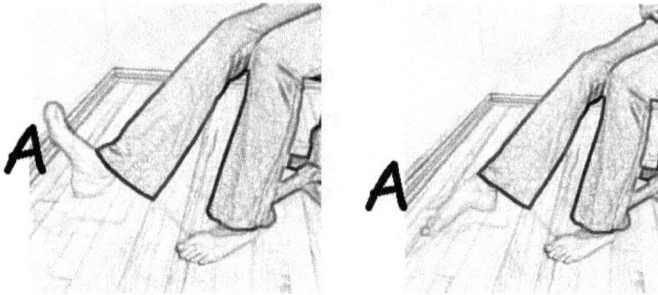

Figure 19-22

If swelling is the cause of your foot pain, this is a great way to help drain the excess fluid out of your lower extremities throughout the day. Simply use your big toe like it is a pen, and draw the alphabet in capital letters in the air from A to Z.

Repeat this with your other foot.

This will cause the ankle to go through the motions of inversion, eversion, plantar flexion, dorsiflexion, and circumduction without having to remember a complicated routine. The motion will cause the lower leg muscles to contract and relax, pumping excess fluid out of the lower extremities back up toward the torso. Circulating those fluids back into the bloodstream means the kidneys will eventually be able to filter out all of the toxic metabolic waste.

This is a great exercise to do to prevent swelling and/or varicose veins.

Legs up a Wall for Lymphatic Drainage

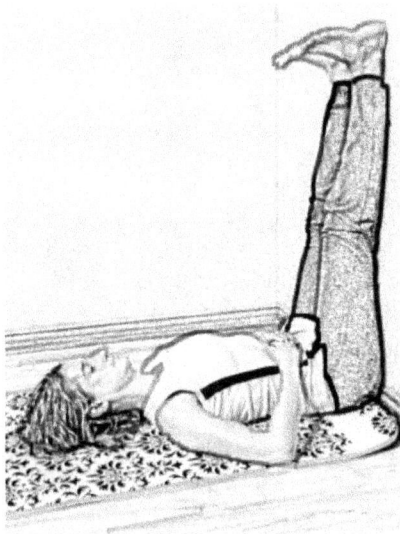

Figure 19-23: Lymphatic Drainage

Another great way to drain the excess lymph from your feet is to rest your legs against a wall. You can also draw the ABCs with your feet like in the previous seated lymphatic drainage exercise to actively milk the lymph out of the most distal tissues of your feet.

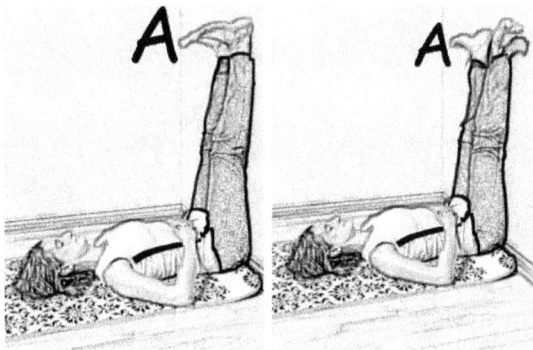

Figure 19-24

Chapter 20: FOOT MASSAGE TECHNIQUES

A FOOT MASSAGE is very beneficial. It gets your muscles to relax, allowing blood to flow and lymph to drain, and it feels good because pressure is taken off sensitive nerves in the lower legs and feet.

Lymphatic Drainage Massage

To drain the lymphatic fluid out of your feet and lower legs, start at the most distal tissues: your toes. Wrap your hands around all of your toes and squeeze to the point you feel good pressure, but not pain (Figure 20-1).

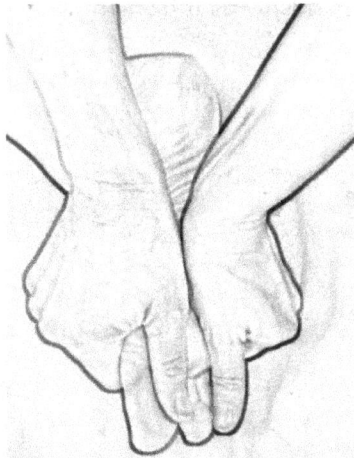

Figure 20-1: Squeezing lymph fluid out of the toes.

Then move your hands up toward the middle of your foot and squeeze again (Figure 20-2).

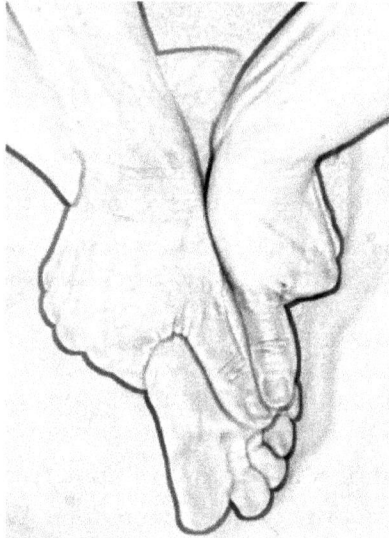

Figure 20-2: Milking the lymph further out of your foot.

Then move your hands to your heel and squeeze. Then squeeze your ankle (Figure 20-3).

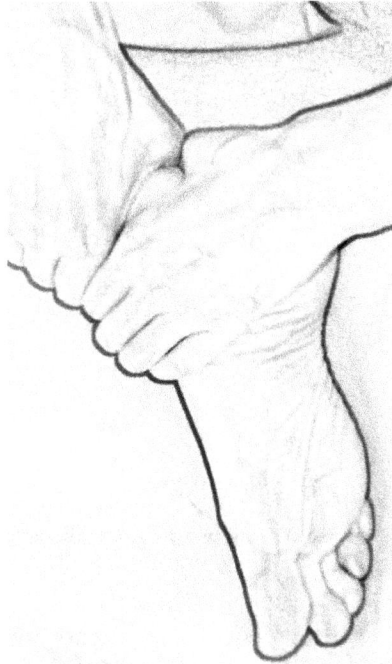

Figure 20-3: Squeezing the lymph out of the ankle.

Then work up your calf muscles, squeezing as you go (Figure 20-4). Pay special attention to the inside of your knees because lymph fluid often gets trapped here (Figure 20-5).

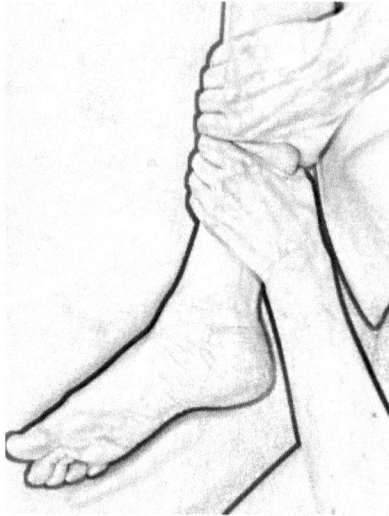

Figure 20-4: Squeezing lymph out of the calf region.

Squeezing the medial aspect of the meaty parts of the knees helps facilitate the lymphatic drainage of the lower extremities. Repeatedly squeezing this region literally milks the excess lymph along the one-way valved vessels.

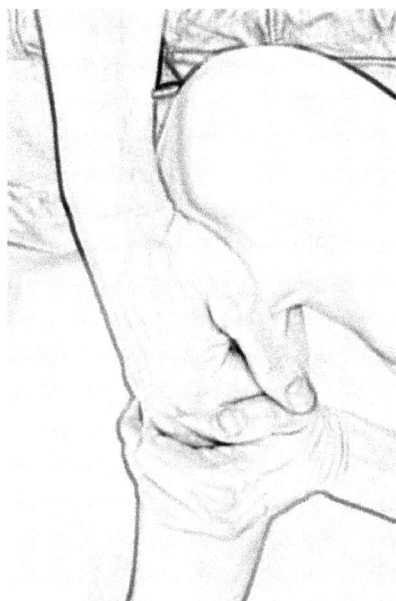

Figure 20-5: Squeezing lymph out of the knee.

I like to use a rolling pin to milk the lymph out of my thighs (Figure 20-6). Thigh muscles are thicker and take more pressure to work out the tightness. I place the rolling pin just above the inside of my knee, press into my inner thigh as I roll the pin up to my groin, and repeat several times.

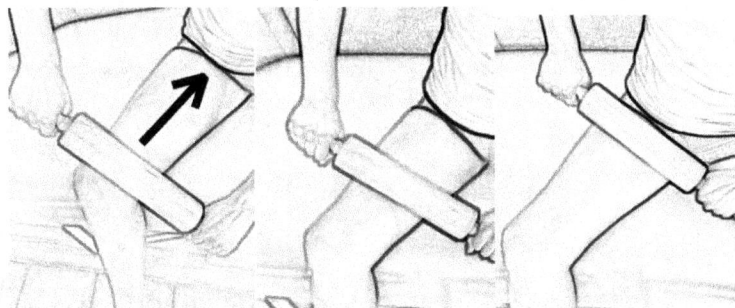

Figure 20-6: Using a rolling pin to milk lymph out of the inner thigh.

I then move the rolling pin to the top of my thigh just above my knee and roll it up the top of my thigh to my hip (Figure 20-7). I repeat this stroking action several times.

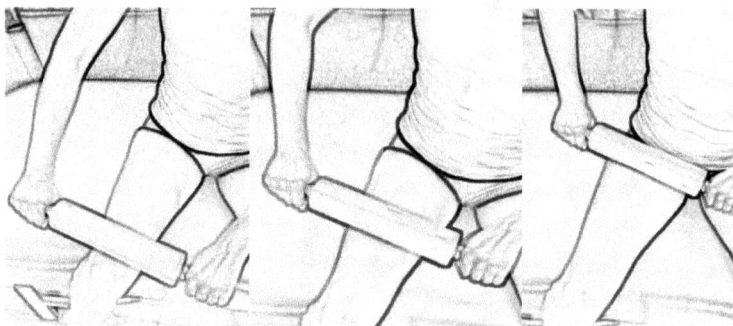

Figure 20-7: Using a rolling pin to drain the lymph out of the top thigh.

Then I roll the rolling pin on the outside of my thigh, knee to hip, several times (Figure 20-8). It is important not to roll back and forth like you would a pie crust, as this would increase the back-flow pressure in the vessels of our leg, increasing our risk of damaging the valves in our veins and lymph vessels, which can lead to varicose veins and swelling of the lower extremities.

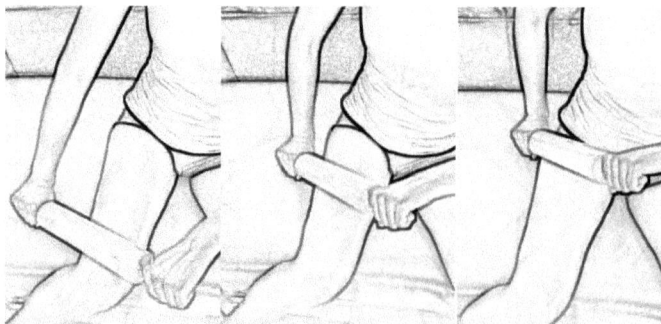

Figure 20-8: Draining the lymph from the outer thigh.

To address the hamstrings, legs up the wall (as in Chapter 19) both stretch and drain the hamstrings. You can also massage the hamstrings by using a foam roller.

Pressure Point Massage for the Feet

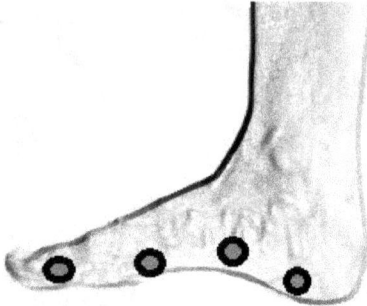

Figure 20-9

To work out any pressure points in your feet (Figure 20-9), start by running your fingers along the arch of your foot and see if you find any tender spots. If you find one, press on it for three breaths and then release. Wiggle your toes to see how it feels. If it feels a little better, repeat the pressure until it feels a lot better (up to three times because you do not want to over-treat and inflame the tissues).

Each time you press on the tender spot, it should be less tender. The tenderness decreases as the excess metabolic waste in the muscle is squished out of the muscle, up the lymphatic vessels toward the heart. The metabolic waste is dumped into the blood stream at the thoracic duct and eventually gets filtered out by your kidneys. If the tenderness does not improve with each squeeze, seek the advice of a massage therapist, chiropractor, and/or physical therapist.

Pressure Points in the Lower Leg

The spots pictured in Figures 20-10 and 20-11 are the locations of common pressure points in the lower leg.

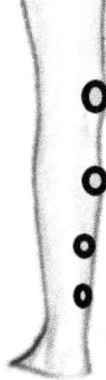

Figure 20-10: Medial and lateral pressure points.

Look for points around your ankles that are tender. Tenderness indicates lymphatic blockage or muscle tension, and tells you that something needs to be worked out. Applying pressure here could potentially alleviate foot pain.

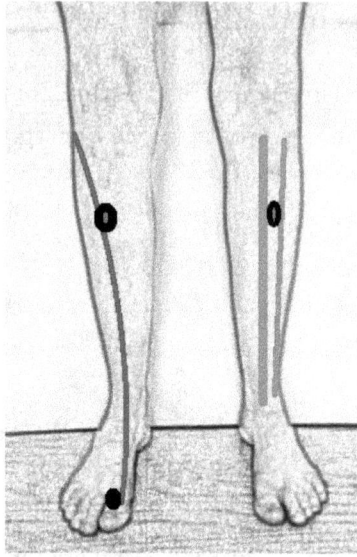

Figure 20-11: Pressure points in the front of the leg.

Then feel the meaty part of the front lower leg between the two long bones (the tibia and fibula; Figure 20-11) and see if you have tender spots there. If you do, press and hold for three breaths to see if this helps your foot pain.

I find that it is better to do frequent, gentle cycles of pressure point therapy than to do intense pressure a few times a week. I teach my patients how to do the therapy themselves so their symptoms do not return between their sessions with me.

Mobilizing Technique

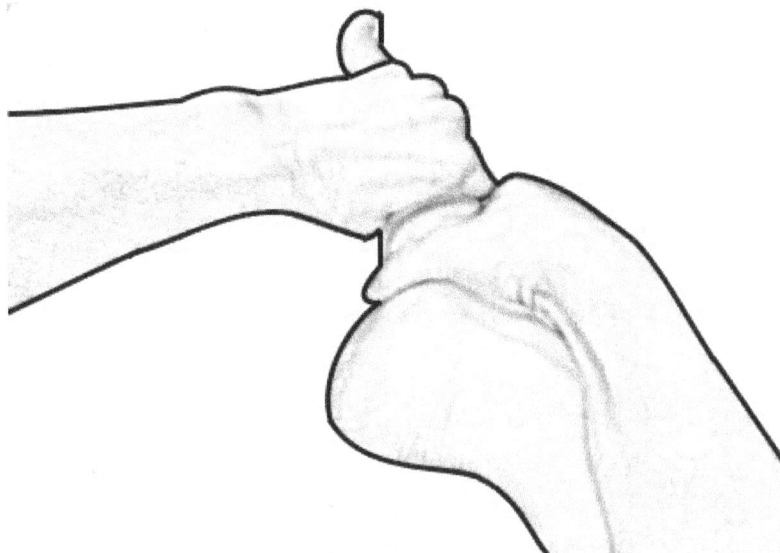

Figure 20-12: Mobilizing the bones in the arches of the foot.

To loosen the tarsal bones of your foot, you can grab your foot as pictured in Figure 20-12. Apply a wringing action (like you are trying to wring out a wet towel). This will loosen your tarsal and metatarsal bones. Moving the bones feeds the joints, wrings out inflammatory metabolic waste, creates space for the nerves, and allows for better lymphatic drainage and blood flow, all of which facilitates healing.

Frequency is more important than intensity or duration because it generally just takes a minute or two to drain the foot of its metabolic waste, but within an hour (if not minutes) it can refill. So take a moment every hour throughout the day to drain your foot of metabolic waste.

Foot Massage Tools

All kinds of foot massaging tools are available to treat foot pain, but you don't have to spend a lot of money on high-tech gadgets.

A cheap massage option is to roll the bottoms of your feet on a golf ball, as shown in Figure 20-13.

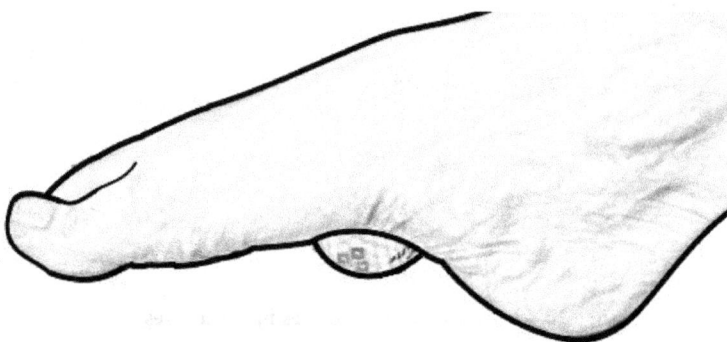

Figure 20-13: Using a golf ball to massage the bottom of the foot.

This works best on carpeted flooring (so the golf ball doesn't shoot out from under the foot). Another option is to put the golf ball in a sock to better control its location under the foot as you roll your foot back and forth on the ball.

Make sure to use enough pressure to massage the muscles, but not so much pressure that you bruise the bottom of your foot.

You can even use an ice cube to massage your feet, or roll your foot on a frozen water bottle as described in Chapter 21.

Chapter 21: ICE OR HEAT THERAPY FOR FOOT PAIN

I F YOU ARE EXPERIENCING PAIN and are looking for an alternative to over-the-counter pain relievers, temperature therapy may be an option. Heat therapy and ice therapy are useful and sometimes can be used interchangeably. Talk with your healthcare provider to see what is best for your individual needs.

Heat Therapy

Heat is a great analgesic (pain reducer) and opens up capillary beds, bringing more blood to the region that is experiencing pain. This is great for tight muscles. However, heat therapy is also inflammatory. If your foot pain is caused by inflammation, heat can make it worse. For example, plantar fasciitis can worsen with the use of heat.

Usually with foot pain, heating the calf muscles is helpful because the inflammation is in the foot, and the muscle spasm pulling on the inflamed tendons is at the foot/heel. So, in general, it is safe to heat your calf muscles when you have foot pain.

Ice Therapy

Like heat, ice is a great analgesic. But ice is also an anti-inflammatory. Ice therapy is a suitable treatment for acute injuries (during the inflamed state) because ice therapy causes your blood vessels to constrict, which reduces blood supply to the region. But if you don't have any inflammation, ice therapy is unhealthy for tissues already starved for blood, as with foot pain that is caused by spastic muscles. This is why I prefer to ice just at the spot of pain on the foot.

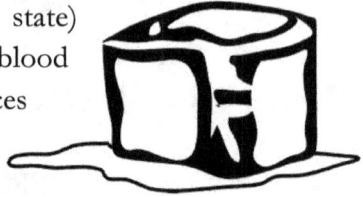

Careful!

Be careful with heat and ice. They are very effective tools when used correctly, but they can be dangerous when used incorrectly or to treat the wrong ailment.

Patients often make an emergency visit to my office after sleeping with a heating pad. This is a dangerous practice. It is too easy to overheat the region and wake up in a terribly inflamed state.

It is also dangerous to sleep with an ice pack, especially if you are on pain pills. I have had more than one patient wake up with frostbite under an ice pack after having slept with one.

The Safest Treatment for Foot Pain

I believe the safest self-treatment for most foot pain is to

1. Heat the lower leg (calf region) for ten minutes to bring nutrient-filled blood to the area and to relax the lower leg muscles.
2. Stretch the calf and foot muscles gently while the muscles are warm and pliable.
3. Finish with two minutes of rubbing an ice cube at the most intense spot of pain in the foot (arch, heel, Achilles) to calm any inflammation that may have worsened with the heat. Note: Wrap half of the ice cube with a cloth so you don't freeze your fingers as you apply the ice (Figure 21-1).

Ice Massage Technique

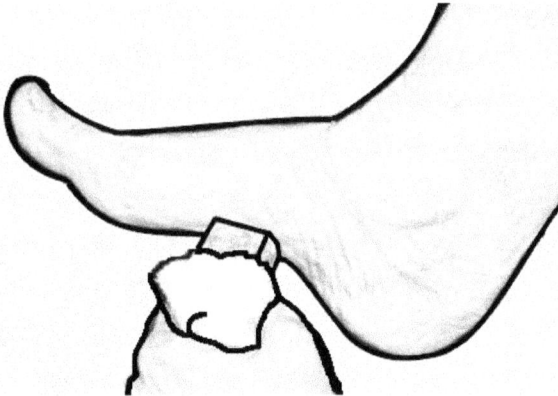

Figure 21-1: Ice massage with an ice cube.

Massaging with ice provides the benefits of pressure relief combined with the cold that constricts your blood vessels.

To massage with ice, wrap half of an ice cube with a cloth (so you don't freeze your fingertips as you apply the ice) and hold the ice to the skin at the region of the most intense pain (Figure 21-1).

You can also apply ice to your feet with a frozen water bottle. Fill a water bottle three-quarters full and put it in the freezer. It can't be full because water can break the bottle as water expands when it freezes.

Once frozen, you can use it to ice massage your foot by rolling your foot on it as in Figure 21-2.

This is a doubly effective technique because it massages and cools the foot at the same time.

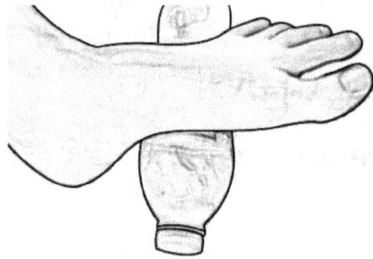

Figure 21-2

Chapter 22: HERBAL REMEDIES AND THERAPEUTIC OILS FOR FOOT PAIN

I F AFTER TRYING ALL of the techniques mentioned in this book to treat your foot pain you still have pain that you cannot get rid of, what next? You'd really like to take a pain pill but know you shouldn't. Instead, try some herbal alternatives. This chapter lists topical remedies, herbal remedies, and therapeutic oils that I have found to be helpful. You can find these at most health food stores, but I recommend asking your healthcare provider what brand they prefer (quality of brands changes over time).

CryoDerm

If your legs, heels or feet are in pain, instead of taking pain pills, think about applying a topical pain reliever. Why take a pill that affects your whole body and potentially harms your organs when a topical provides localized relief without the negative side effects of oral medication?

My favorite it CryoDerm. It is a cooling blend of menthol, arnica, and other herbs.

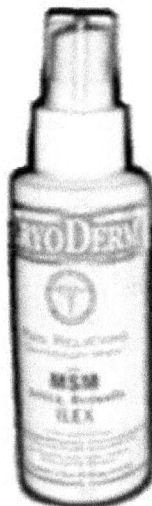

It comes in a spray, roll-on, and gel applications.

I prefer the spray for the foot. The spray is the easiest form of application. You simply spray it on the affected region, making sure to point it toward the foot and away from your eyes. CryoDerm is painful in the eyes, and if it comes in contact with the eyes, it needs to be thoroughly rinsed out.

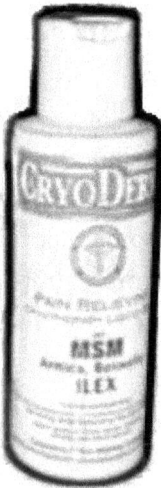

The gel form requires you to rub it in, making your hands feel the cool effect where it is not needed. The gel form is great for multiple-person use. I use the gel and spray when applying CryoDerm to my patients.

I don't like using the roll-on application for the feet because the feet tend to be dirty, making it necessary to clean the feet before every application of the roll-on. If you don't clean your feet, you contaminate the roller. The roll-on is great for cleaner regions, like the neck, because you can massage the CryoDerm in with the roller without getting CryoDerm on your hands or risk accidently getting over-spray of the CryoDerm in your eyes.

CryoDerm is available on Amazon and some chiropractic offices.

White Willow Bark for Pain

White willow bark is the natural version of aspirin. Pharmacological companies discovered the active ingredient in white willow bark that decreased pain, and now they chemically produce it in a concentrated form. If aspirin were developed today, it would be labeled as a prescription drug because its lethal dose is so minuscule.

White willow bark contains aspirin in its natural state and is less likely to irritate the stomach lining or cause death. It is more expensive than a bottle of aspirin, but if you adhere to the lifestyle changes this book suggests, you should not need much of this herbal remedy. White willow bark is available on Amazon.

Kava Kava Root for Muscle Tension

Kava Kava root is a natural muscle relaxer. It may help take the edge off of foot pain caused by tense muscles or if you suffer from leg and/or foot cramps. Available on Amazon.

Caution!

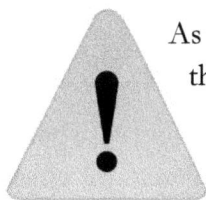

As with any muscle relaxer, you should first try these remedies when you don't have to drive, work, or do anything that you would not do while impaired. It is best to take these herbs at night to help you relax and sleep.

Other Herbs That May Help

Other herbs that may help with your foot pain are curcumin (a natural anti-inflammatory from turmeric that is best absorbed with pepper) and bromelain (a pineapple enzyme, another natural anti-inflammatory). I would not advise using these herbs without guidance from a practitioner who is well versed in herbal remedies.

Therapeutic Oils That May Help

Essential Oil of Peppermint for Muscle Aches

Essential oil of peppermint is good for tense muscles. It has a nice cooling effect, which also helps diminish aches in the muscle. Massage three to four drops of peppermint oil into the foot and/or calf muscles.

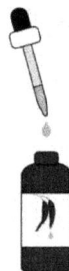

Essential Oil of Clove for Muscle Tension

Essential oil of clove is also good for muscle tension. Clove has a nice warming effect, which helps relax tense muscles. Massage three to four drops of clove oil into the foot and/or calf muscles.

Essential Oil of Cypress for Edema

Essential oil of cypress reduces swelling, which can cause pain and limit healing. Massage a drop or two of cypress oil onto the regions that are swollen (the calf muscles, the arches, and/or knees).

My Advice on Using Natural Remedies

You can seek advice from a naturopath or another health practitioner who is well versed in herbs to find out if other herbal remedies would be better for your specific needs. However, like prescription medication, I am not a fan of relying on a surplus of pills, tinctures, etc. Natural or not, such treatments should be used sparingly so they work when you need them.

Chapter 23: WHY SEE A CHIROPRACTOR FOR YOUR FOOT PAIN?

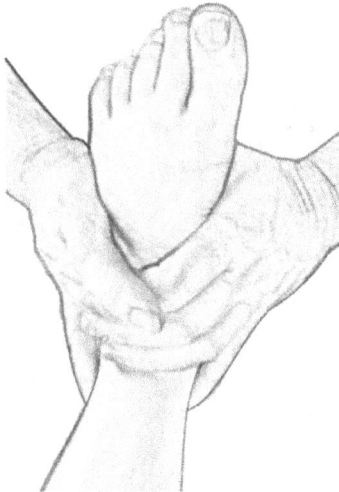

Figure 23-1: Foot adjustment.

CHIROPRACTORS are primary care physicians who complete just as many years of education as an allopathic medical doctor. They are more than just neck and back doctors who manipulate (adjust) spines. They are also educated on joints of the extremities such as feet, ankles, knees, and hips. So if you suffer from foot pain, they will not just address your feet, but also look at how your pain might be affecting your knees, hips, pelvis, and spine.

It only takes months to learn how to adjust, but it takes years to learn how to properly diagnose and determine treatments (dietary, herbal, home care, physical therapy, etc.). It also takes years of study to learn when not to treat, refer a patient to another doctor, and know which specialist to refer to.

Chiropractors complete more hours of education in anatomy, orthopedic imaging, and nutrition than medical doctors do.[4] They have about the same hours in differential diagnostics.

A medical doctor's education is filled with pharmacology because their primary form of treatment is prescribing medication. This approach often just removes or glosses over symptoms instead of dealing with the underlying causes of illness or pain.

Primary care physicians who deliver babies (obstetricians) are, in fact, trained surgeons and often depend on surgical interventions instead of seeking less invasive responses to maintain a healthy pregnancy. Chiropractors study pharmacology and surgery only minimally because they aim to help you achieve wellness without invasive treatments.

However, chiropractors are able to help you determine if more invasive treatments are needed and will refer you to specialists accordingly.

What Is a Chiropractic Adjustment?

---

[4] Jensen, "Chiropractic Education vs. Medical Education."

During a chiropractic adjustment (also called a manipulation), a chiropractor applies a high-velocity, short-lever arm thrust to a bone to decompress a joint, restoring normal motion to the joint and/or normal alignment of the bones. Let me explain in layman's terms how a chiropractor does an adjustment.

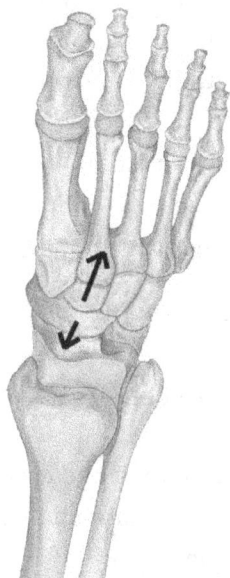

To perform an adjustment, the chiropractor introduces a quick stretch to the muscles surrounding a joint while staying within the joint's normal range of motion.

When the bones are quickly (yet shallowly) moved apart during an adjustment, the barometric pressure of the fluid within the joint decreases. As with any fluid, decreasing the pressure causes gases to be released (in this case, oxygen, nitrogen, and carbon dioxide).

An everyday example of this phenomenon is when you open a can of soda. The soda in the can is under pressure, and when you open it, the pressure on the fluid decreases, and bubbles come out of the liquid. A joint, however, is a closed "container," so the "bubble(s)" pop immediately.

Why an Adjustment Helps

Many things occur during an adjustment, and they all happen almost simultaneously.

First, the chiropractor introduces a quick stretch to the muscles surrounding a joint. When the nerves feel this quick stretch, they reflexively make the muscles relax to protect the muscles from tearing.

There is no risk of a chiropractic adjustment tearing muscles because the stretch doesn't go deep enough to cause harm, but your nerves and muscles don't know this. All they know is that an external force is making the muscles stretch quickly, so the nerves protect the muscles from such external forces. Therefore, an adjustment causes spastic muscles to reflexively relax. The now-relaxed muscles help keep the joint mobile and functional, allowing it to heal.

Healing Occurs Even at a Biochemical Level

During an adjustment, other biochemical reactions occur. The body releases endorphins into the area of the adjustment. This provides the short-term pain relief people report after an adjustment. The long-term effects of an adjustment are faster healing and restored full range of motion.

Joint Manipulation Is so Much More Than Just a Stretch

I gave many massages before becoming a chiropractor, and I will never forget giving my first neck adjustment a couple of decades ago. The poor patient had torticollis (a stiff, spastic neck). It would have taken me more than an hour of massage to get that neck to relax and partially mobilize. Yet one quick adjustment and that patient, in one millisecond, felt more relief than I could have given him with hours of massage therapy alone.

During an adjustment, a chiropractor moves a joint within its full healthy range of motion. It is safe because the chiropractor is far from overstretching the ligaments.

If you do not move enough, your joints degenerate. When is the last time you stretched all of your joints to their full range of motion? There is a reason we say, "If you don't use it, you lose it." People stiffen as they get older not because of their chronological age, but because of their lack of stretching over time. Look at yogis. There are 100-year-old yogis who are more flexible than average middle-aged Americans.

I like to say that chiropractic manipulations are like going to a partner yoga class, but with a skilled partner who knows how to get to the end range of all your joints quickly and safely. Chiropractic adjustment is like yoga with an "oomph."

Simply moving joints helps them heal (Figure 23-1). Joints need motion to be fed with nutrients and to have their waste materials removed.

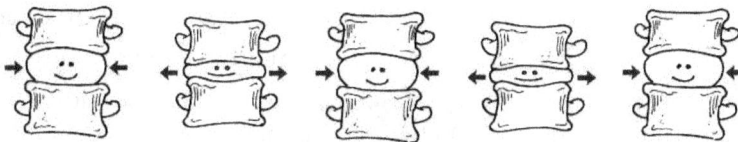

Figure 23-2: Happy joints being fed by movement.

When you sit or stand still for too long, the weight of your body slowly squishes the fluid out of your joints (Figure 23-2). Your joints become deficient of the much-needed nutrients that would normally flow into a healthy, moving joint. If you sit too long, you literally starve your joints, causing them to degenerate over time.

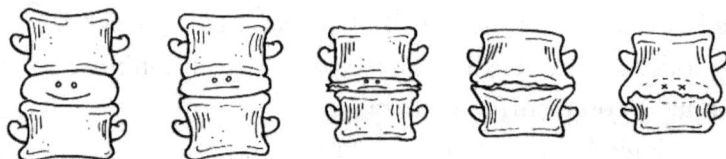

Figure 23-3: Discs degenerate over time because of a lack of movement.

These effects are not limited to the spine; they can occur in any joint in the body. The poor joints of the feet not only bear the weight of the whole body, but they also are the first ones to strike the ground when you move around. This repetitive strain and pressure causes joints to degenerate over time.

Don't Blame Age for Your Degenerating Joints!

Bones and joints are not rods of iron that rust with time. They are living tissue that degenerates with abnormal stressors over time. Everyday activities result in micro trauma to tissues (Figure 23-4). As you age, your ability to heal slows down, so you feel your body slowly lose the battle of healing.

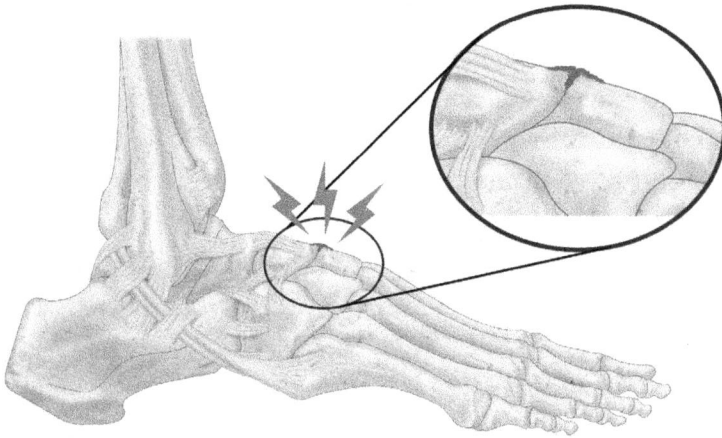

Figure 23-4: Thickening of tarsal bones in response to micro trauma from repetitive stressors.

When you are young, you heal rapidly because the joints are plump with nutrient-filled fluid, which is why you do not feel this micro trauma occurring. As you age, each of these injuries is felt more profoundly because you take longer to heal and the micro traumas begin to accumulate. This results in degeneration and arthritic changes (Figure 23-4).

You can't blame your age for bunions and hammer toes. They are a result of being hard on your feet over time. Yes, some people are more genetically prone to these conditions, but being good to your feet will help you not only prevent these conditions from developing, but also help your feet improve instead of worsen over time!

Even young adults who do not move enough will experience degeneration in their joints. I am seeing people at younger ages getting degenerative joint disease from sitting too much from a very young age.

Like physical movement, an adjustment literally "feeds" the joints it moves. When the gas bubbles form in the joint and pop, the fluid stirs (Figure 23-5). Nutrients flow in, facilitating the joint's healing and reversing the degenerative process.

Chiropractic Adjustment

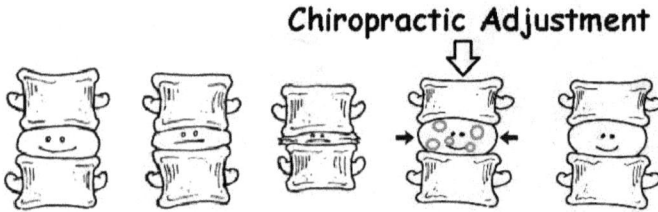

Figure 23-5: Chiropractic adjustment decompresses a joint, reversing the degenerative process.

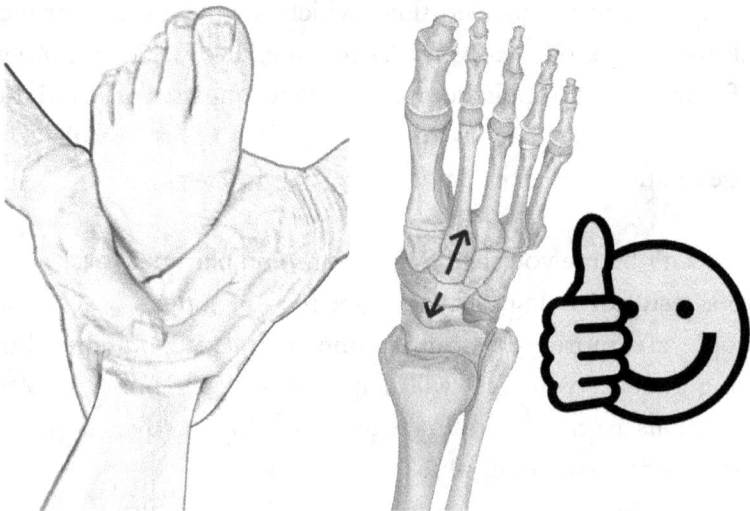

Figure 23-6: Foot adjustment

Popping Your Fingers and Toes Prevents (Not Causes) Arthritis!

When you see your chiropractor, they should also pop your fingers and toes. The idea that popping your fingers and toes was bad because would lead to arthritis is an old wives' tale.

Research has found that those who pop their fingers and toes were less likely to develop arthritis over time.[5] Again, popping joints is good for them!

Now I am not endorsing over-adjusting joints. I wouldn't pop your joints every twenty minutes. My rule of thumb is, if you pop a joint and feel relief for hours, that's great. If you pop a joint but feel the need to pop the joint again within an hour, you did something wrong. If you truly corrected the problem, the relief would have lasted longer. If the relief is short lived, you are just experiencing the endorphic relief that occurs with an adjustment (which typically lasts less than an hour). If you are finding yourself self-popping many times a day, see a chiropractor for a professional adjustment. After which you should find yourself not needing to pop yourself as often.

Even Chiropractic Side Effects Are Beneficial

The health benefits of an adjustment are often greater than expected. By stretching the vertebrae of the spine apart, more space is created for the nerves that exit the spinal cord. Nerves don't like pressure, and they function better with space.

---

[5] deWeber, et al. "Knuckle Cracking and Hand Osteoarthritis," *Journal of the American Board.*

Results on Our Internal Organs

Chiropractic positively affects internal organs by decreasing pressure on the nerves that supply these organs, improving blood flow to these organs and lymphatic drainage from these organs.

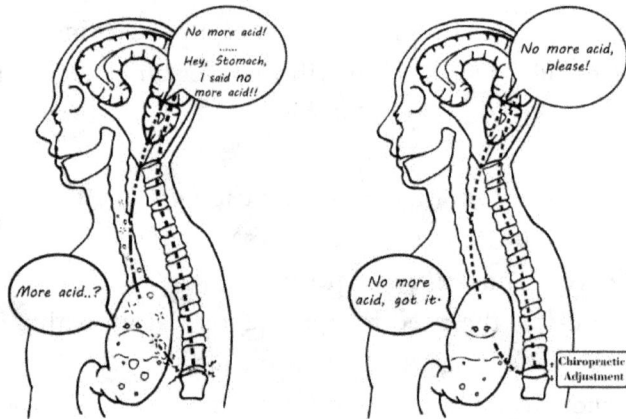

Figure 23-7: Nerve irritation negatively impacting the stomach followed by relief with chiropractic manipulation

Chiropractic manipulation frees the nerves between the nerves of any pressure or irritation. Such pressure or irritation impairs the flow of information between the body and the brain (like how a radio has more static when there is interference between your radio and the radio station). Once free of such static, the brain and body are able to "hear" each other clearly. Better communication between the mind and body makes for better functioning organs, leading to a healthier body in general. This is why I love chiropractic.

Chiropractic care for more than just pain relief

Chiropractic works not only for foot and leg pain, but for general wellness. Chiropractic adjustments restore mobility and space to the spine, and chiropractors educate patients on healthy lifestyle habits to reduce the cause of their symptoms.

Nerves that exit the neck region supply the head and upper extremities. After treating neck pain, I often hear things like, "I haven't had a migraine since," "My sinuses have cleared," and "My vertigo is gone!"

Nerves that exit the mid-back region send signals to the organs in the mid-torso, including the lungs, stomach, spleen, and liver. After treating for mid-back pain, I have heard things like "My asthma is better" and "My GERD has improved" (Figure 23-7).

Nerves that exit the lower back region of the spine send signals to the organs in the lower torso, including the lower intestines, reproductive organs, and lower extremities. After treating low back pain, I often hear things like, "My foot pain is better," "My bowel movements have been more regular than ever," "My menstrual cycle is more normal," "My ED seems to have resolved," "I thought I was infertile, and now I am pregnant!"

After treating children, their parents report, "They are calmer," "They are sleeping better," and "They are able to focus more."

I prefer these types of "side effects" to the side effects people experience with allopathic medicine, which often has incredibly long lists of possible negative side effects, including "Can cause death." When you take any medicine, there is

177

always some negative effect; sometimes your body can tolerate it, but sometimes the negative effect causes enough harm that it ends up outweighing the benefit.

Side effects of medications can lead to foot pain because the drug's toxicity often affects the tissues farthest from the body's main organs the most.

Despite what uninformed people may believe, there is little mystery about why chiropractic works. Its effectiveness and efficiency have been scientifically studied for decades.[6]

I look forward to a time when patients try chiropractic first to see if it can help (knowing their chiropractor will send them to a medical doctor or surgeon if they feel their condition is inappropriate for chiropractic care).

Even if chiropractic doesn't end up helping you with your foot symptoms, you can always fall back on the medical route. But if you start with the medical route, especially surgery, sometimes there is no turning back. I believe if people saw a chiropractor first, it would solve a lot of our healthcare problems in America (both the costs of healthcare and the general health of this country). Cost of care initiated with a

---

[6] Bryans, et al., "Evidence-based Guidelines for the Chiropractic Treatment of Adults with Headache," *Journal of Manipulative and Physiological Therapeutics*; Astin and Ernst, "The Effectiveness of Spinal Manipulation," *Cephalalgia;* University of Maryland Medical Center, "Migraine headaches"; Bronfort, et al., "Effectiveness of Manual Therapies," *Chiropractic & Osteopathy*; Haas et al., "Dose-Response and Efficacy of Spinal Manipulation," *Spine Journal.*

doctor of chiropractic often is less than treatment initiated with a medical doctor.[7]

But let's get back to our topic...

Don't think that allopathic doctors and chiropractors are the only people who can help you with your foot pain. Other providers you can seek treatments from are acupuncturists, podiatrists, massage therapists, and doctors of osteopathy.

---

[7] Liliedahl et al., "Cost of Care for Common Back Pain Conditions Initiated with Chiropractic Doctor Vs Medical Doctor/Doctor of Osteopathy as First Physician: Experience of one Tennessee-based general health insurer," *Journal of Manipulative and Physiological Therapeutics.*

Chapter 24: PROFESSIONAL MASSAGE TOOLS FOR FOOT PAIN

T HERE ARE MANY TECHNIQUES for massaging the feet. Most massage therapists use their hands to massage out tension in the muscles of the feet and body. Some use tools like hot stones to take advantage of the softening effect heat has on muscles. If you have foot pain from inflammation, make sure to let your feet cool after any treatment that involves heat (as discussed in Chapter 21).

Cupping

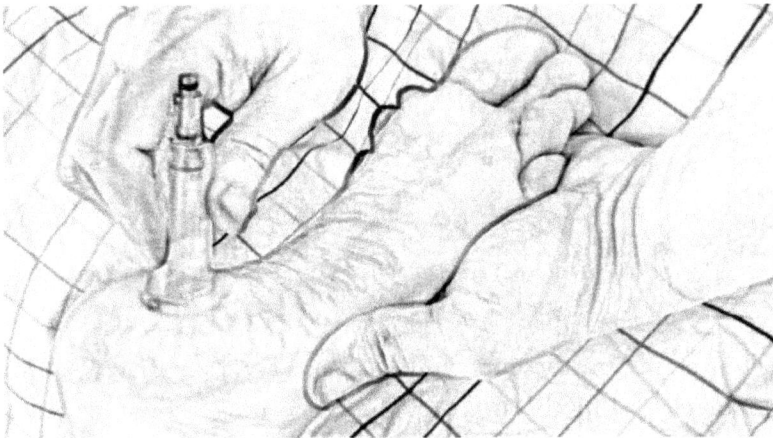

Figure 24-1: Cupping being done on my low back.

If you've seen large, perfectly round discolorations on an athlete's skin, you've seen the outward signs of cupping.

Cupping involves creating negative pressure on tissues. A therapist uses a cup to create a vacuum that draws the skin up and away from the muscles (Figure 24-1). This is the opposite of negative pressure used during a regular massage, where the practitioner physically presses on the tissue to push out the metabolic waste and break up adhesions.

There are a variety of ways to create negative pressure with cupping. Glass cups are usually used because they are durable and easy to sanitize. Different sized cups are used for different sized muscles and different applications (Figure 24-2).

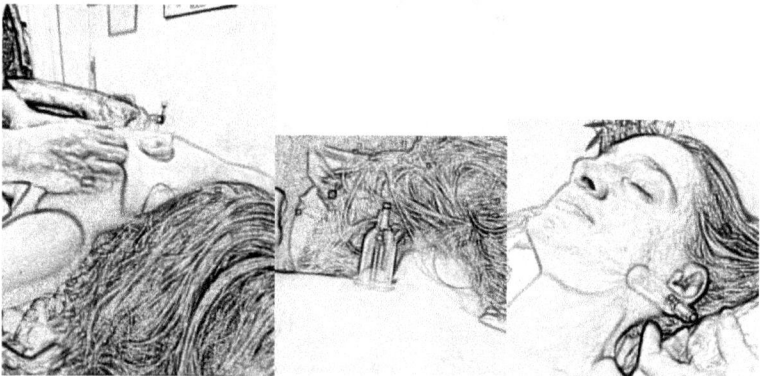

Figure 24-2: Different sizes of cups are used for different regions.

The vacuum in the cup can be created a variety of ways. One involves heating the air inside the glass cup and then placing it on a trigger point or acupressure point. As the air cools, it creates a vacuum, and the skin gets drawn up into the cup. A newer technique uses a pump to suck the air out of the cup to create a vacuum, as shown in Figure 24-3.

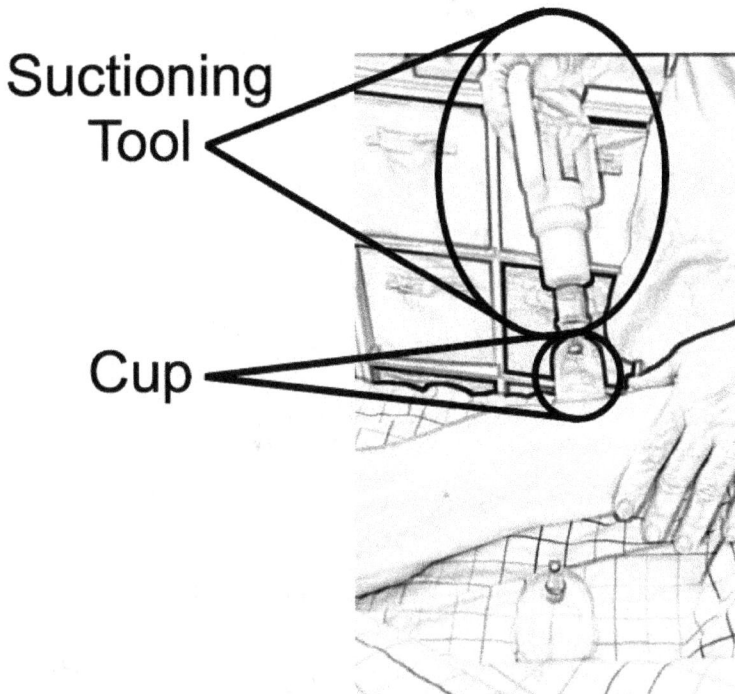

Suctioning Tool

Cup

Figure 24-3: Cupping using a suctioning tool and the cup

As the skin gets sucked into the cup (Figure 24-4), the skin layer separates from the muscle layer, breaking up adhesions in the fascia. Leaving the cup at these points for a few minutes brings more blood to these tissues. As a result, the tissues heal, and their function improves.

Leaving a cup on a spot for too long can cause bruising or blistering, so be sure to communicate to your practitioner if the cups are getting uncomfortable.

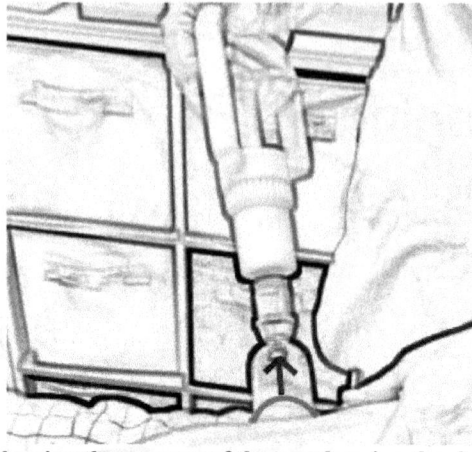

Figure 24-4: Showing the vacuum of the cup drawing the skin up and away from the calf muscle, bringing more blood to the region, facilitating healing.

A New Application for This Ancient Tool

Some massage therapists use cups as a massage tool. They apply oil to the skin first so they can glide the cup over a region (Figure 24-5). This type of massage is a negative pressure massage. Unlike a regular massage, in which positive pressure squishes metabolic waste out of the muscles, a massage therapist can use the negative pressure of the cup to milk metabolic waste out of the region by gliding the cup over it.

You may prefer this negative massage to a deep-tissue (positive) massage when your tissues are too tender to handle pressure. Some find this technique more comfortable. Some prefer positive pressure. The only way to know which you prefer is to try each and decide for yourself which feels more comfortable and effective for you.

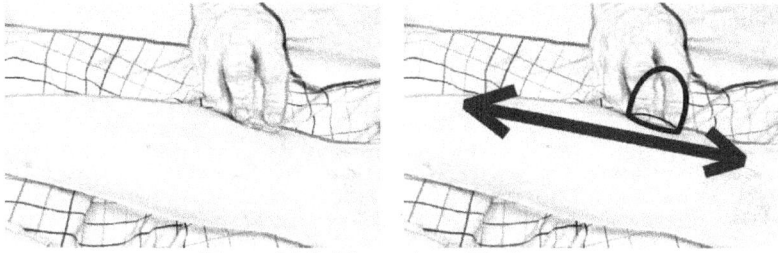

Figure 24-5: Massaging with the cup.

Usually, cupping results in reddening of the skin. I believe that if you bruise heavily afterward, the practitioner used too much suction. More is not always better. Bruising is a sign of tissue damage, not healing, but sometimes a little bruising is unavoidable. When cupping is done well, bruising should be minimal, and the reddening of the skin should fade within a few days.

Blue = Bruising = Bad

☹

Fading = Facilitated Healing = Fabulous

☺

What causes this reddening of the skin?

Every cell naturally produces lactic acid as a waste product. Muscles and skin contain significant amounts of blood vessels that drain waste from and bring nutrients to their tissues. But the fascia (connective tissue) between the skin and muscles does not contain a lot of blood vessels. Lactic acid can build up in this layer and irritate the nerves, resulting in pain.

Cupping releases the toxic lactic acid from the fascia, facilitating healing. Another way to release this toxic metabolic waste is through an ancient Asian technique, Gua Sha.

Gua Sha: Using a Soup Spoon or Shell as a Massage Tool

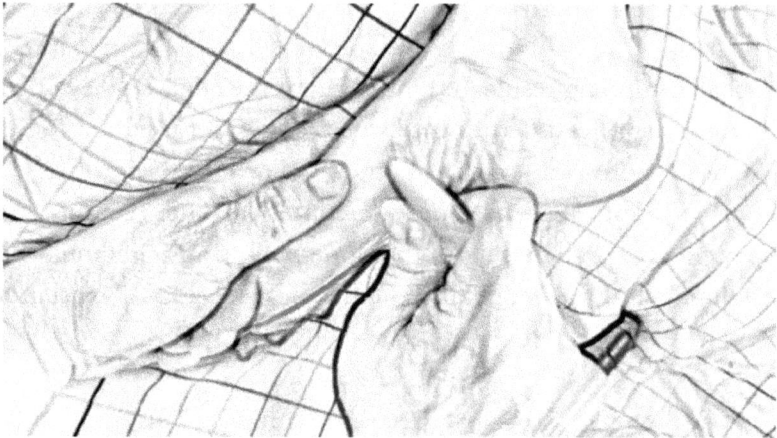

Figure 24-6: Foot massage using a smoothed-out shell

Gua Sha is another treatment that releases the toxic lactic acid from the fascia, facilitating healing. The skin reddens as a hard object like a soup spoon or a smoothed-out shell (as in Figure 24-6), rubs back and forth, breaking up scar tissue. Again, this reddening of the skin is not bruising because it does not turn blue (a bruise results when tissue is filled with blood that lacks oxygen, turning the skin blue); the redness diminishes over two to five days (unlike a bruise, which can take more than five days to fade).

Often the calf muscles will be released with Gua Sha to take pressure off the structures in the foot and alleviate foot pain.

Some physical therapists use a modernized version of Gua Sha called Graston where they use a metal tool instead of a Chinese soupspoon or shell.

In the hands of a skilled practitioner, either tool can be used effectively. It's not the tool that determines the effectiveness of the treatment, but the one wielding the tool

If there is scar tissue in the foot, I prefer to use Rapid Release Technology to break up the adhesions because it is less painful than undergoing Gua Sha. I am so impressed by Rapid Release Technology I gave it its own chapter.

Chapter 25: RAPID RELEASE TECHNOLOGY

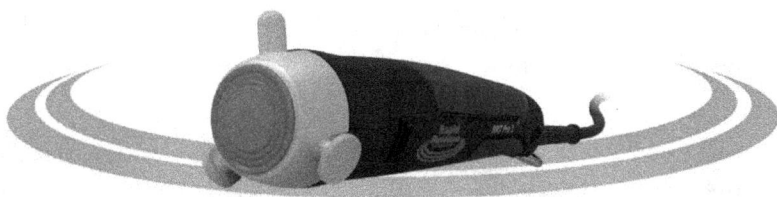

I FIND THE Rapid Release Technology (RRT) great for treating conditions like plantar fasciitis, heel spurs, bursitis, and nerve pain. The only downfall is that it often is very ticklish to vibrate the bottom of the foot! Personally, I would rather be tickled than tortured with scraping techniques like Gua Sha on the bottom of my feet.

Using Technology to Break Up Adhesions

When your body heals itself, it forms adhesions. Adhesions are stiff, ropey fibers that pull on healthy tissues. They can even pull on organs, disrupting their function. Adhesions can also impair blood flow and lymphatic drainage and pinch nerves. Because adhesions seriously impair the body's ability to function well, they must be broken up.

The Rapid Release Technology device works in two ways. It vibrates, which closes the pain gates in nerves, dulling pain; and it percusses, which breaks up adhesions that form during the healing process. When you place the tool's head on the skin, you can see a circular wave traveling from the head through the skin's fascia. (Fascia is long, thin tissue that covers underlying tissues; it also encloses muscles.)

In unhealthy tissue (tissue that has abnormal adhesions or scar tissue), the circular wave is small or nonexistent because the thick fibers of the adhesions don't move as freely as healthy, flexible tissue fibers. As the adhesions "melt" and break up, the circular wave becomes more pronounced and expands outward—physical evidence that the device is breaking up the fibers that were laid down abnormally.

Good for More Than Just Foot Pain

I have had patients who responded amazingly well to the Rapid Release Technology. It's a great modality, especially when patients are in an acute state. Even if they can't tolerate light touch, patients easily tolerate the RRT's high speed and short stroke. The combination of vigorous yet gentle treatment gives patients immediate relaxation of the acute spasms and improved range of motion.

Their muscles relax, their pain diminishes, and their ailments heal faster.

Diagnosing Tiny Fractures and Breaks

I also use the Rapid Release Technology to help rule out fractures. If a bone has even a hairline fracture, vibrating it will often cause searing pain.

This is especially useful for toes that often get stubbed on the corners of furniture and ankles that roll! Such injuries can swell so badly and be so painful that it is difficult to tell if the bones are cracked. Even X-rays can miss fresh fractures, because an X-ray is a two-dimensional view of a three-dimensional object. Cracks without separation are easily missed with such imaging.

In such cases, I use the RRT to see if the vibration feels good or painful. As you can imagine, powerful vibration feels awful on a bone with a crack in it.

To learn more about the Rapid Release Technology, check out http://rapidreleasetech.com.

Chapter 26: KINESIO TAPE FOR FOOT PAIN

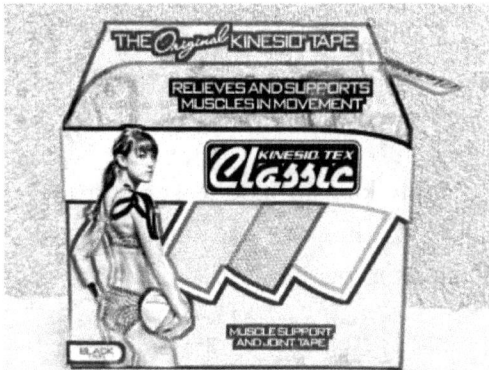

Figure 26-1: Kinesio Tape

KINESIO TAPE has helped me as well as many of my patients reduce pain while working out, participating in strenuous activities, and otherwise pushing our muscles to their limits. Some people claim kinesio tape only works because of the placebo effect. I say even if this is the only reason it works, I will take a placebo over any toxic chemical any day, as long as it works without harm.[8]

Kinesio tape is a short, flexible cloth tape that is worn to relieve muscle pain or to encourage muscles to work more efficiently.

---

[8] Williams et al., "Kinesio Taping," *Sports Medicine.*

Kinesio tape helps massage muscles as they move. With the proper application, the tape stretches and compresses, then relaxes with the body's movement, lowering the pressure. This pumping action aids in blood flow and lymphatic drainage, which facilitates healing.

It can also aid in the alignment of the body while it is in motion; for example, it can be applied to tug on the shoulders when they begin to slouch.

Kinesio Tape for Foot Conditions

You can also apply kinesio tape to support the arches of the foot (Figure 26-2), helping the alignment of the foot to facilitate healing from plantar fasciitis, ankle sprains, and more.

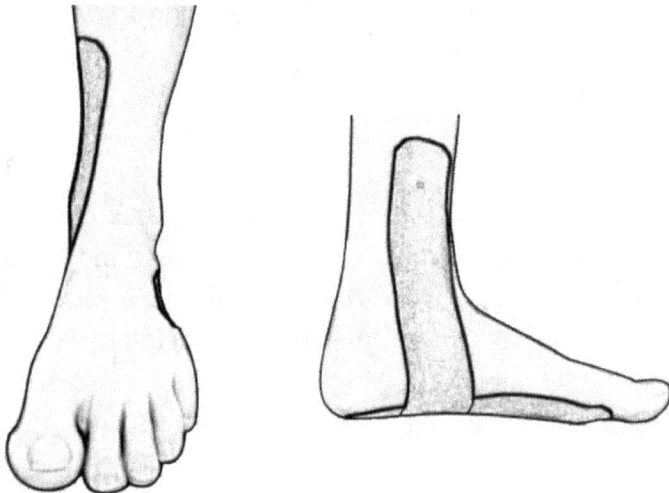

Figure 26-2: Kinesio Tape Supporting the Longitudinal Arch

You can apply kinesio tape to the heel and calf regions of the foot to facilitate feeling from posterior heel spurs and Achilles tendonitis (Figure 26-3).

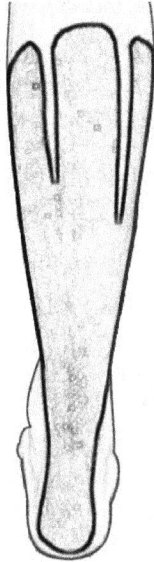

Figure 26-3: Kinesio Tape Supporting the Achilles Tendon

You can apply kinesio tape to the bottom of the foot (Figure 26-4). This helps drain the inflammatory proteins that cause the pain of plantar fasciitis, facilitating healing.

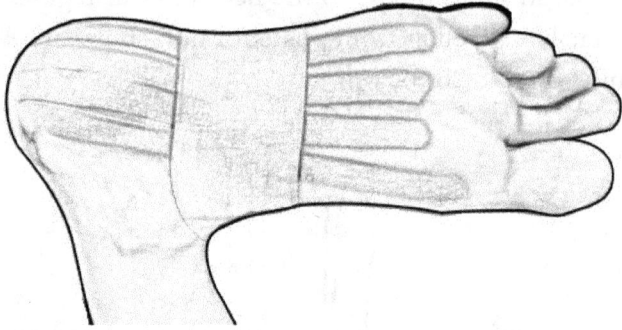

Figure 26-4: Kinesio tape on the bottom of the foot to support the plantar fascia

Kinesio tape does no harm, is not expensive, and usually helps. This is why, despite the lack of strong scientific support, I have enough clinical anecdotal evidence to use it in my clinic.

Chapter 27: ACUPUNCTURE FOR FOOT PAIN

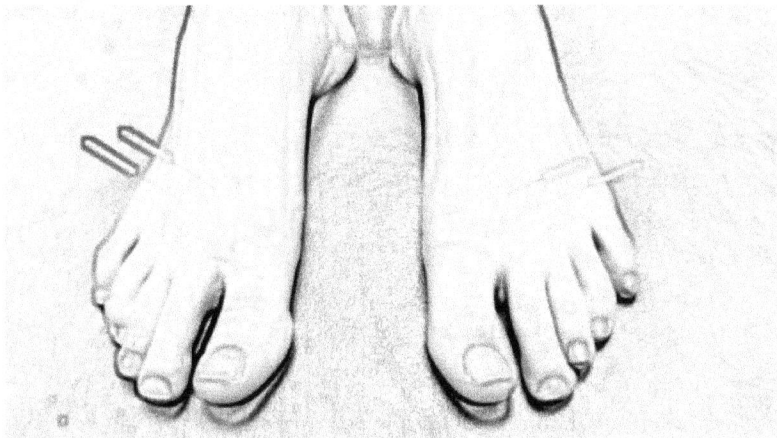

Figure 27-1: Acupuncture for foot pain.

YOU MAY BE hesitant to try acupuncture to treat your foot pain, or you may be fearful of having needles stuck into your muscles. I have a phobia of needles myself, yet acupuncture does not bother me. It helps that the needles are tiny and they do not inject or draw anything from my body.

You barely feel most of the needles. I will admit, some needles may go into a tender spot. For me, I find the spots at the base of my first and second toes very sensitive to needles.

Remember, if the area is too tender, you can have the practitioner remove the needle. You can always try that spot again at a future appointment. As your health improves, fewer and fewer spots should be tender.

If you find most of the needles uncomfortable, you can ask the practitioner to use smaller needles. After my whiplash injury, I could barely handle the tiniest of needles. Some needles are so tiny that you should not be able to feel them at all. I knew I was improving as the needles became painless and I was able to use larger needles with each subsequent visit.

I encourage you to read the following Q&A with my acupuncturist to understand what acupuncture is and how it may be able to help.

Interview with Jennifer Stone, BS, LAc

When I decided to start seeing an acupuncturist, I chose Jennifer Stone, BS, LAc, because I had heard that she is not only a great acupuncturist, but a famous one! Her research has furthered her profession, and she has been an instructor for acupuncture.

Because many people are unfamiliar with acupuncture, I asked Jen to explain the procedure.

What Is Acupuncture?

Acupuncture is a procedure in which fine needles are inserted into specific points on the body to relieve pain and promote homeostasis. Acupuncture originated in China and is the result of more than four thousand years of empirical evidence. Acupuncture has been shown to be an effective treatment for twenty-eight diseases, symptoms, or conditions.[9]

What Schooling/Licensure Is Required?

A licensed acupuncturist requires three years of postgraduate training for a master's degree and two additional years for a Doctor of Oriental Medicine degree.

Most states require NCCAOM (National Certification Commission for Acupuncture and Oriental Medicine) board certification to receive a license. Some states allow MDs and chiropractors to practice acupuncture with two hundred to three hundred hours of acupuncture training.

How Does Acupuncture Work?

When an acupuncture needle is inserted into the skin, the body reacts, blood flow increases, and a variety of chemicals are released that reduce inflammation, stop pain, and promote healing.

Are There Side Effects?

---

[9] World Health Organization, "Acupuncture: Review and Analysis"; Stone and Johnstone, "Mechanisms of Action for Acupuncture," *Current Treatment Options in Oncology.*

Sometimes patients have mild bruising or itching at the needle site. Occasionally someone will faint.

Are There Different Types of Acupuncture?

Yes. Traditional Chinese medicine (TCM), Japanese meridian style, auricular (ear) acupuncture, five element style, and Korean style are commonly practiced in the United States.

How Is Acupuncture Different Than a Physical Therapist's Dry Needling?

There is no difference. Dry needling is acupuncture, and acupuncture needles are used. The company that began marketing dry needling training to physical therapists invented the term. The training is as little as twelve hours with no clean needle technique training and is not accredited.

Is Acupuncture Safe?

Yes. A review of acupuncture for low back pain reported that out of 7,161 people, no serious adverse events associated with the acupuncture were reported.[10]

This last question brought up an important point. If you are going to try a treatment, be it acupuncture, chiropractic, or something else, make sure the practitioner is not only properly

---

[10] Taylor-Swanson and Stone "Acupuncture for Low Back Pain."

accredited, but has a good reputation. If a patient is hurt during a treatment, don't blame the tool or technique; instead, question the ability of the one yielding the tool or performing the technique.

So how do you go about finding a healthcare provider? I explain that in the next chapter.

Chapter 28: WHAT TO LOOK FOR IN A PRACTITIONER

HOW DO YOU find a group of healers (be it a chiropractor, medical doctor, massage therapist, physical therapist, osteopath, naturopath, acupuncturist, or any other type of healer) to help you treat your foot pain? This is a loaded question, but the following are my two cents of advice.

First, find your practitioners by asking friends and family for referrals. The internet is a good place to find out more about a practitioner, but it is not the best place to choose one. Anyone can look good online and post fake testimonials. Try to use sites like www.yelp.com where people can post good and bad reviews without the business owners cherry-picking only the good reviews. This will increase the likelihood of getting legitimate evaluations.

Try to find people who have seen the specific practitioner you're considering and ask them about their experience. When you find a practitioner you think you want to work with, ask yourself the following questions.

Does the Practitioner Really Listen to Me?

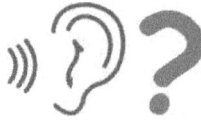

Sadly, many in the medical field are in it for the wrong reason, or their reasons do not match your needs. You need to find a practitioner who has a passion for helping their patients. One indicator of this is how well they listen to their patients during an appointment. Most proper diagnoses come from taking an accurate history and getting a complete description of the current symptoms. Most physical examinations, imaging, and laboratory work are performed to verify the diagnosis, not to find the problem.

Unfortunately, many doctors get burned out because of the fiasco that is the current political and insurance landscape. They are forced to see more people in less time and are required to complete more paperwork and coding of a patient's symptoms. Eventually, many practitioners end up shutting down emotionally, closing off their humanity in order to survive everything that is expected of them.

Doctors are people too, but you should not place the doctor's needs above your own when seeking treatment. Find a doctor whom you like on a personal level and who genuinely seems to care for you. This will positively affect your healing.

Does the Practitioner Give Me the Time I Need?

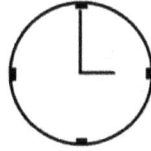

Understand that more time does not necessarily mean a greater quality of care. If the practitioner is efficient and very good, they will not need as much time, but you should feel like you are receiving their full attention and a full treatment when you are with them. You should feel that you got what you needed. I always end my treatments by asking my patients if I took care of everything, or if there is something else they need. This assures me I covered what they came in for, and if I did not, this gives the patient the opportunity to express their needs.

Sometimes I just need a few minutes to treat a patient; other times I end up spending a whole hour. It makes scheduling tough, but the rare times my patients have to wait, they know it wasn't because I overbooked, but because someone needed more time. My patients appreciate that I give extra time if needed, and they recognize that someday it may be they who need that extra time.

Can the Practitioner Help Me? How Many Treatments Will it Take? How Much Will it Cost?

Ask the practitioner at the beginning whether your aliment is something they understand, have experience with, and have had success treating. What do they think your prognosis is?

Specifically for foot pain, ask if they can provide orthotics, manipulations, kinesio tape, topical pain relief, etc. A practitioner is limited by the tools in their belt, so make sure they have a wide variety of tools to attack your foot pain with!

Ask if they will be able to get you well within a reasonable budget? If the treatment is costly, maybe you can find a less costly fix while still maintaining the quality of care. Costlier does not necessarily mean higher quality care. Beware, however, that you sometimes get what you pay for. Do not shortchange the quality of your healthcare to the point of negatively affecting the quality of your care.

If the practitioner does not think you have a good prognosis, find a different practitioner. If your prognosis is bad, that is simply an opinion of someone who has not routinely seen success with your ailment. Find a different practitioner, one who has had success with your ailment, so they can give you a better prognosis.

If people are going to spend their health dollars on a treatment, that treatment should have a favorable outcome. To help determine whether progress is being made, measurements should be taken incrementally during the course of the treatments to show objectively whether the patient is responding favorably. If there is no measurable improvement partway through the treatment, then the condition needs to be reexamined. You may be getting treatment for the wrong condition. You cannot keep doing the same treatment and expect a different result.

I have had multiple patients come see me after their previous chiropractor failed to make them feel better after dozens of treatments. I was glad these patients were willing to suspend blame on the tool of chiropractic. With my chiropractic skills, I was able to help them feel better after just a few treatments. The rare times I cannot help a patient, I direct them to health practitioners who can.

It is important to find a practitioner who is willing and able to be your partner in obtaining optimal health. That practitioner should know their limitations and whether the treatment options for you go beyond their abilities. If they are not willing to be your partner, they are unlikely to help you reach optimal health. When a practitioner reaches their limitation in being able to help you, that is their limitation, not necessarily your limitation on being able to get well.

Think of all the aliments that used to be considered untreatable. They were not truly untreatable, but instead were outside the abilities of medical care at the time. These same ailments *are* treatable today because of the increase in medical knowledge. Unfortunately, we healthcare providers may not know the treatment you need, even if a treatment is currently available for you.

It reminds me of the old joke, "Do you know what they call the person who graduated at the bottom of his class at medical school? Doctor." Just because one doctor or one type of healthcare practitioner cannot help you solve your problem does not mean your problem is unsolvable.

Is the Practitioner Open to Me Seeing Other Practitioners?

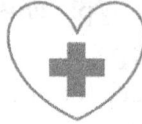

I always welcome other practitioner's views on my patients' wellness. Not just from specialists in other fields, but from other chiropractors as well. Everyone brings something unique to the table, and sometimes new eyes bring new perspectives. I have a dozen patients who see other chiropractors for treatments I do not offer or because the other chiropractor is more convenient (closer to their work or home); these patients see me only when their treatments are not helping as expected and they need another opinion. Some patients simply like to have a relationship with multiple chiropractors so they are more likely to be seen in a timely manner.

I encourage all of my patients to see a variety of other health practitioners (medical doctors, acupuncturists, massage therapists, physical therapists, etc.). At a minimum, these other practitioners confirm my diagnosis and treatments. If they do not confirm it, then it prompts me to reexamine the problem more deeply. This can provide a learning experience for me and further confirmation for the patient. Or the patient may have two different opinions and more information to bring to a third practitioner to find the root of the problem. In either case, the collaboration is more helpful than the Lone Ranger approach.

I cannot tell you how many times patients have come to me after seeing several doctors, each of whom gave the patient a different diagnosis. I examine the patient and review what has already been done so I can help them determine the root cause and they can figure out their next step toward wellness.

My least favorite thing is when a patient comes in with what I call a "garbage can diagnosis," which is basically a fancy combination of Latin words that describe their symptoms but not any underlying causes or conditions. Then, armed with this "diagnosis," a medical doctor will generally attempt to cover up the patient's symptoms with drugs. It is relatively easy to do, and everyone is happy at the cessation of symptoms. But the long-term cost of this approach is immeasurable: The patient's health will continue to deteriorate over time because no one is addressing the root of the problem.

To make matters worse, the effectiveness of any medicine decreases over time as the body learns to break it down. This reduced effectiveness results in having to increase the dose over time. Sadly, the patient is trained to blame this problem on the fact that they are aging. No! The patient needs to learn what the root of the problem is so they can properly treat it and so their body can start healing over time instead of worsening.

I love my job. Every day I get to watch people transform from the belief that their health was naturally going to worsen with time to a place where their lives and abilities actually *improve* over time. I have many patients that are healthier in their forties and fifties than they were in their twenties and thirties.

If you receive satisfactory answers to the first four questions, then after seeing the provider, ask yourself the following questions:

Is the Practitioner Actually Helping Me?

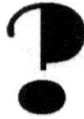

?

Do their treatments hurt? Some therapists have a "no pain, no gain" mentality, resulting in treatments that may be more painful than they need to be.

If you feel like your healthcare provider (be it massage or physical therapist, chiropractor, acupuncturist, or any other practitioner) is hurting you, even if they are not, your belief that they are hurting you will impair your healing. This phenomenon is called "the negative placebo effect."

I always tell my patients to listen to their instincts. If what I do or say does not jive with them, they should tell me. Their instinct always trumps my recommendation or technique. It just means we have to find another technique that works for them, both physically and mentally. You cannot separate the two.

Many of my patients say that, for such a small female, I give a mighty adjustment and dig deep with my soft-tissue work. But many patients receive ultra-gentle care from me. I tailor my treatment to the patient's needs and limitations. I am not going to adjust a construction worker the same way I would an elderly lady with osteopenia.

There are times where I am pressing on tender muscles, but I aim to produce good pain. My patients understand that it may hurt in the moment, but the body knows it is a good hurt and a productive movement toward wellness. I never want to cause bad pain. That, to me, is a pressure that causes more harm than good, such as bruising healthy tissues. I aim to mobilize joints, not strain them.

This is where the art of practice comes into play. Anyone can move a joint, but not everyone can move it safely and well in a manner that that patient is comfortable with. That is why such practices take years of education and requires licensure.

Is the Practitioner Living Up to My Expectations?

At your first appointment, a practitioner should give you a rough timeline of when you should start seeing results. If you are not seeing the results as expected, get another opinion. Do not be afraid to seek more than one healer's advice to validate the root cause of your pain.

When a patient isn't seeing results as expected, it can be due to the provider not treating you completely or a misdiagnosis resulting in the wrong treatment being prescribed.

You have the right to see as many healing professionals as you need to in order to get to the core of your condition. Each type of practitioner (and maybe even each individual practitioner) will have their own individual technique that they can bring to the table. If nothing else, they can help verify that you are receiving the right kind of treatment.

Good luck creating your optimal healing team!

Chapter 29: GOOD PRACTICES FOR HEALTHY FEET

Triad of Wellness for Healthy Feet

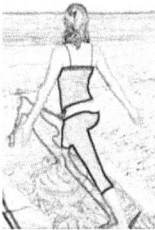

Sleep & Think Well
Relax & meditate
to rest and heal well

Support with good
shoes or orthotics,
compression socks,
gel cushions or
stabilize with splints
or a boot

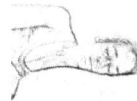

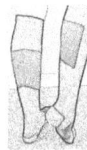

Exercise & Stretch Well
Check your posture, stretch, &
strengthen regulary.
Invert frequently to help
the drainage of
blood flow and lymph.

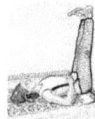

Eat & Hydrate Well
Provide nutrients to every cell in
your body, and hydrate your
muscles so they don't cramp!

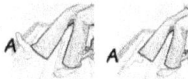

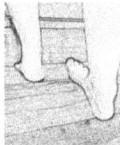

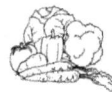

Chapter 30: RECAPPING THE TOP SEVEN WAYS TO COMBAT FOOT PAIN

TO SUMMARIZE MY ADVICE IN THIS BOOK, the top seven ways to combat foot pain are:

1. Wear quality supportive shoes (with orthotics if needed).
2. Rest as needed (wear a foot brace or boot if needed).
3. Heat tight muscles and ice inflamed tissue.
4. Do exercises and stretches for the foot and legs.
5. Avoid masking your symptoms with drugs (fix the root problem).
6. Eat healthy (real) food, and drink enough water (to help tissues heal and prevent cramps).
7. Surround yourself with a team of health professionals.

I hope this book has been informative, enabling you to be more collaborative with your professional healthcare providers, so you can create a lifestyle that leads to happy feet and a happy life.

Wishing you wellness,

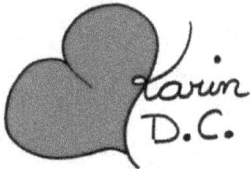

Karin Drummond, DC

If you liked this book, or if it has helped you or a
loved one with their foot pain,
please let me know by
writing a review on **Amazon.**

Thank you!

Review of
Exercises & Stretches
for Foot Pain

Strong and flexible muscles in the foot,
lower leg and thighs for better foot health:

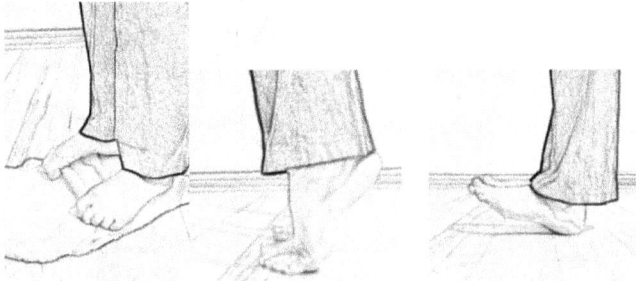

Figures 19-1 & 19-2: Strengthening the muscles of the
bottom of the feet, back of the lower legs and front of the
lower legs

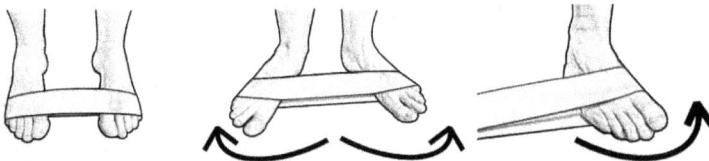

Figures 19-3 & 19-4: Strengthening the muscles of the
sides of the legs

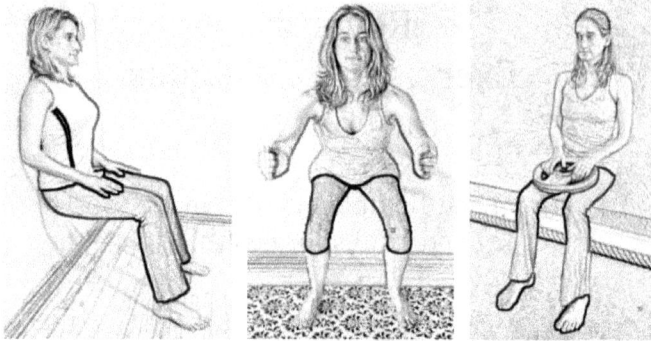

Figures 19-5 to 19-8: Strengthening the muscles in the front of the thighs

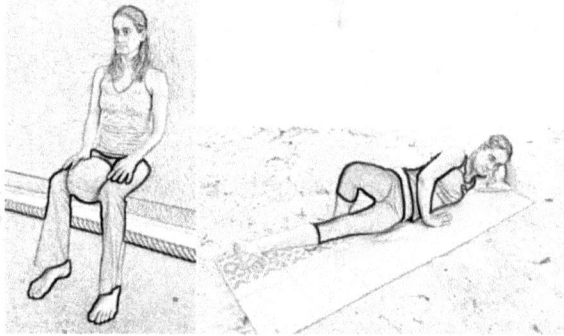

Figure 19-9 & 19-11: Strengthening the inside thigh muscles

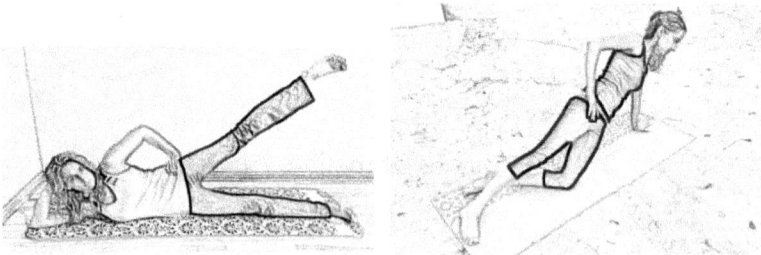

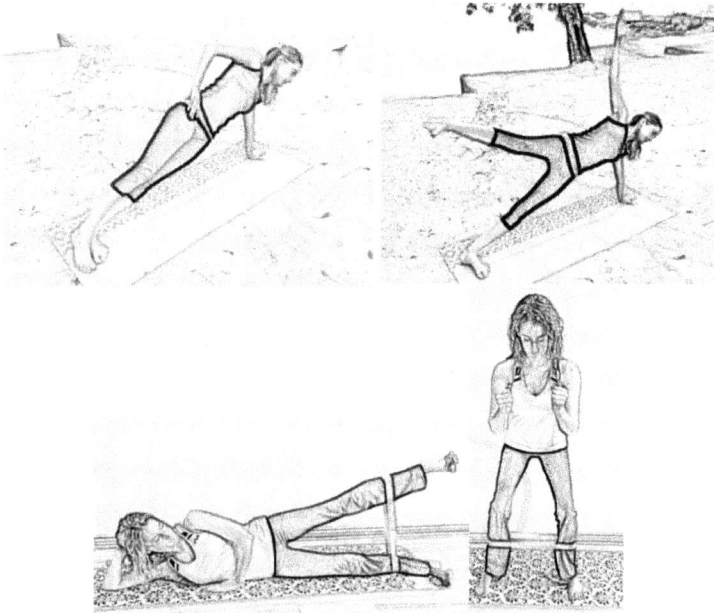

Figures 19-12 to 19-18: Strengthening the outside muscles of the thigh

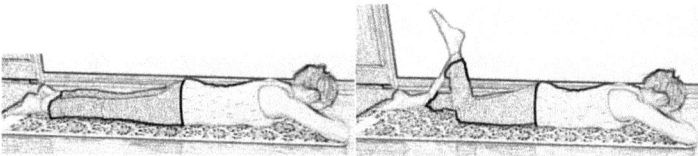

Figures 19-19: Strengthening the backside muscles of the thigh (hamstrings)

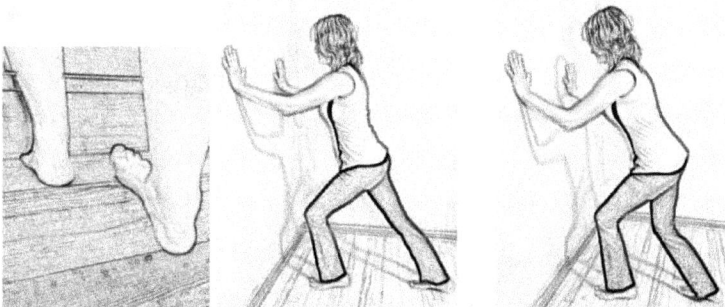

Figures 19-20 & 19-21: Stretching the calf muscles

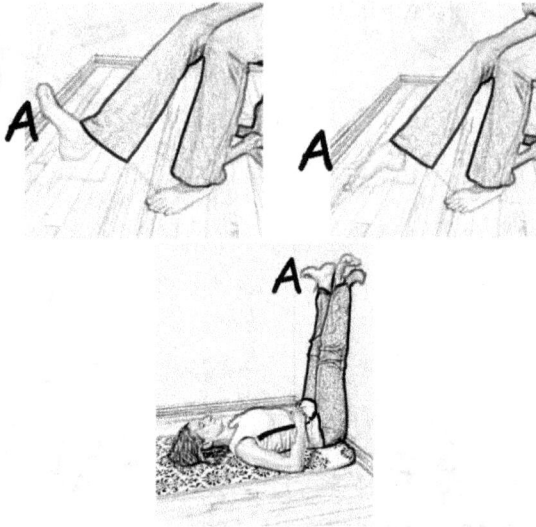

Figures 19-22 &19-23: Draining lymph out of the lower
extremities

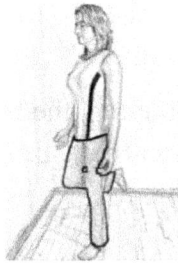

Figures 18-1: Strengthening proprioception

REFERENCES

American Gastroenterological Association. "Study Shows Long-term Use of NSAIDs Causes Severe Intestinal Damage." ScienceDaily. www.sciencedaily.com/releases/2005/01/050111123706.htm.

Astin, J.A. and E. Ernst. "The Effectiveness of Spinal Manipulation for the Treatment of Headache Disorders: A systematic review of randomized clinical trials." *Cephalalgia* 22, no. 8 (2002): 617–623.

Bronfort, G., M. Haas, R. Evans, B. Leininger, and J. Triano. "Effectiveness of Manual Therapies: The UK evidence report." *Chiropractic & Osteopathy* 18, no. 3 (2010). doi:10.1186/1746-1340-18-3.

Bryans, R., M. Descarreaux, M. Duranleau, H. Marcoux, B. Potter, R. Ruegg, L. Shaw, R. Watkin, and E. White. "Evidence-based Guidelines for the Chiropractic Treatment of Adults with Headache." *Journal of Manipulative and Physiological Therapeutics* 34, no. 5 (June 2011): 274-89. doi:10.1016/j.jmpt.2011.04.008.

deWeber, K., M. Olszewski, and R. Ortolano. "Knuckle Cracking and Hand Osteoarthritis." *Journal of the American Board of Family Medicine* 24, no. 2 (2011): 169–174. doi:10.3122/jabfm.2011.02.100156

Haas M., D. Vavrek, D. Peterson, N. Polissar, and M.B. Neradilek. "Dose-Response and Efficacy of Spinal Manipulation for Care of Chronic Low Back Pain: A randomized controlled trial." *Spine Journal* 14, no. 7 (2014): 1106-1116. doi:10.1016/j.spinee.2013.07.468.

Jensen. P. Your Chiropractic Wellness (blog). "Chiropractic Education vs. Medical Education." http://yourchiropracticwellness.com/tag/chiropractic-education-vs-medical-education.

Liliedahl, R.L., M.D. Finch, D.V. Axene, and C.M. Goertz. "Cost of Care for Common Back Pain Conditions Initiated with Chiropractic Doctor vs Medical Doctor/Doctor of Osteopathy as First Physician: Experience of one Tennessee-based general health insurer." *Journal of Manipulative and Physiological Therapeutics* 33, no. 9 (2010): 640–643. doi:10.1016/j.jmpt.2010.08.018.

Stone, J.A.M. and P.A.S. Johnstone. "Mechanisms of Action for Acupuncture in the Oncology Setting." *Current Treatment Options in Oncology* 11, no. 3 (2010): 118–127. doi:10.1007/s11864-010-0128-y.

Taylor-Swanson, L.J. and J.A. Stone. "Acupuncture for Low Back Pain: A systematic review of randomized controlled trials." Prepared for the Washington State Bureau of Labor and Industries. September, 2016.

University of Maryland Medical Center. "Migraine headaches." Last reviewed September 29, 2015. http://umm.edu/health/medical/altmed/condition/migraine-headache#ixzz3axxDHytg.

Vicodin Addiction. "Nearly 100 Percent of the World's Vicodin Prescriptions Are Used in U.S." www.addictionvicodin.com/addiction-news/all-the-worlds-vicodin-prescriptions-in-united-states/.

Williams, S., C. Whatman, P.A. Hume, and K. Sheerin. "Kinesio Taping in Treatment and Prevention of Sports Injuries: A Meta-Analysis of the Evidence for its Effectiveness." *Sports Medicine* 42, no. 2 (February 2012): 153–164. doi:10.2165/11594960-000000000-00000.

World Health Organization. "Acupuncture: Review and Analysis of Reports on Controlled Clinical Trials." http://apps.who.int/medicinedocs/pdf/s4926e/s4926e.pdf.

Zimmerman, H.J. "Drugs Used to Treat Rheumatic and Musculospastic Disease." In *Hepatotoxicity: The Adverse Effects of Drugs and Other Chemicals on the Liver,* 2nd ed. Philadelphia: Lippincott, 1999, 517–553.

ABOUT THE AUTHOR

Karin Drummond, DC, lives in Bloomington, Indiana. She graduated with distinction from the University of Victoria with a bachelor of science degree. She finished the four-year doctorate of chiropractic degree at the University of Western States in 2000. She moved to her husband's hometown of Bloomington, Indiana, and has practiced there ever since. She now calls it home, living at its edge in the country with her husband and two children. She has been voted her town's number one chiropractor seven times as of 2016.

Passionate about living well, she keeps up with new research in the health field and practices what she preaches. Her patients have told her for years that she needed to write a book because she is such a great source of information on healthy living. Once she discovered how easy it was to publish a book, she decided to take advantage of this medium to help spread her thoughts on living well. Her first book, *Top Seven Ways to Combat the Effects of Sitting,* was published in 2015 and was a finalist in the 2016 Best Book Awards in the Health: Diet and Exercise category. She has published several books since then, and she is planning on publishing many more books on a variety of topics.

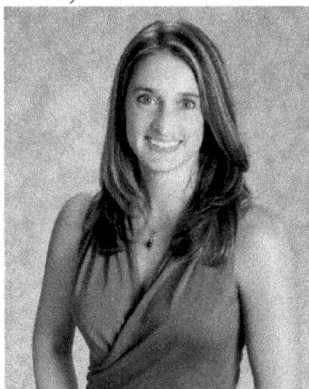

www.drummondchiropractic.com

Other Books by Dr. Karin Drummond

Available now:

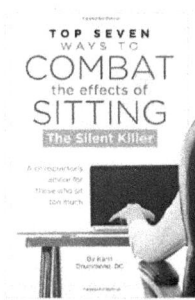

Top Seven Ways to Combat the Effects of Sitting: The Silent Killer
Finalist in the Best Book Awards in 2016 in the Health: Diet and Exercise category.
A must-read for those who sit too much.

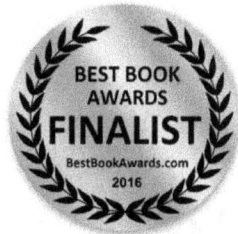

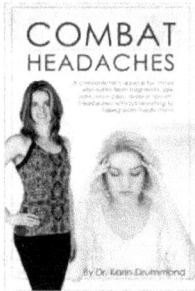

Combat Headaches
For those who suffer from migraines, jaw pain, sinus pain, and/or tension headaches without resorting to taking pain medication.

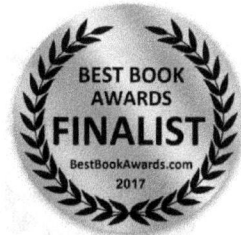

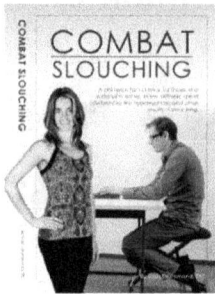

Combat Slouching

For those who suffer from aches, pains, stiffness, spinal deformities like hyperkyphosis, and other effects of slouching.

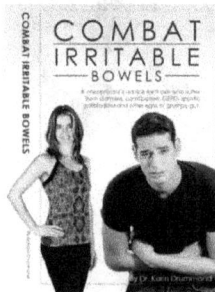

Combat Irritable Bowels

For those who suffer from diarrhea, constipation, spastic gallbladder, inflammation of the bowels, and other causes of abdominal pain.

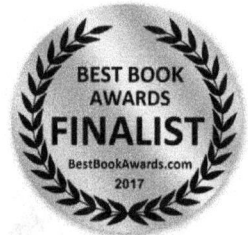

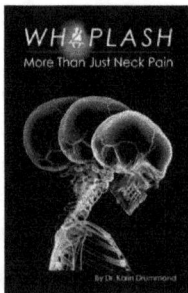

Whiplash: More Than Just Neck Pain

This booklet explains some of the mechanisms of whiplash and symptoms to watch out for.

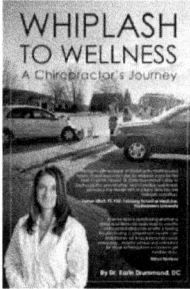

Whiplash to Wellness: A Chiropractor's Journey

The whiplash patient can easily relate to Dr. Karin Drummond's denial of the severity of symptoms and the frustration of daily life after this type of injury. We benefit from her journey as she shares her gems of knowledge. In true Dr. Drummond fashion, she speaks to us with compassion and knowledge, and educates us on modalities of recovery.

–Dr. Lisa Robinson, MD, Joie de Vivre Medical

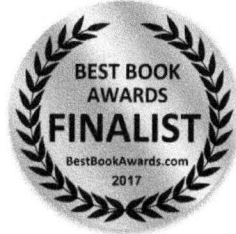

Combat Jaw Pain

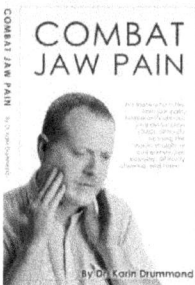

For those who suffer from jaw pain, temporomandibular joint dysfunction (TMD), difficulty opening the mouth straight or completely, jaw popping, difficulty chewing, and more.

Combat Neck Pain

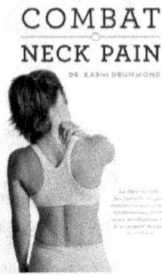

For those who suffer from torticollis, whiplash, degenerative cervical spine, disc herniations, pinched nerves, muscle spasms, and other causes of neck pain and stiffness.

Combat Low Back Pain

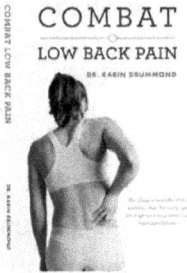

For those who suffer from sciatica, disc herniations, back spasms, and other low back conditions.

Coming soon:

Combat Insomnia

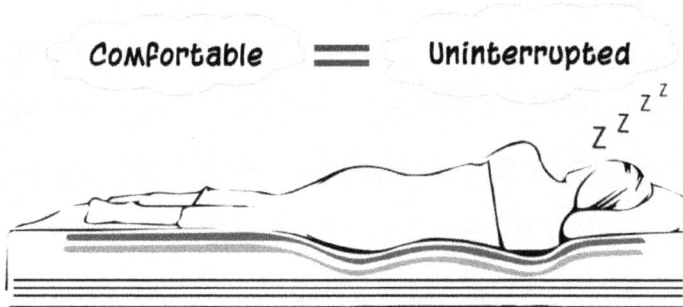

Comfortable == Uninterrupted

No more tossing & turning at night

and many other books…
All to help you find your personal path to wellness.

To find out more, visit Dr. Karin's website:
www.drkarindc.com

or Drummond Chiropractic's website:
www.drummondchiropractic.com

www.ingramcontent.com/pod-product-compliance
Lightning Source LLC
Chambersburg PA
CBHW072126270326
41931CB00010B/1686